Renal Diet Cookbook

The Complete Low Potassium, Low-Sodium Guide for 2000 Days of Easy and Delicious Kidney's Recipes

BONUS 30-Day Meal Plan for living a healthy life

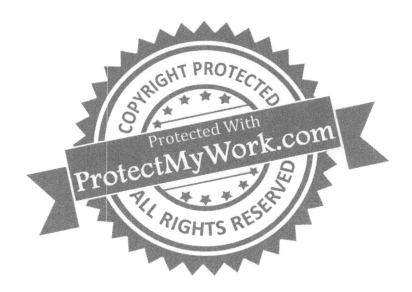

Contents

Introduction

People with poor kidney function must adhere to a renal or kidney diet in order to lower the amount of waste in their blood. Blood contains leftovers from meals and drinks that have been ingested. When renal function is compromised, the kidneys are unable to filter or remove waste as they should. If waste is allowed to remain in the blood, the patient's electrolyte balances can suffer. A diet that is friendly to the kidneys can sustain healthy kidney function and delay the onset of kidney failure. A renal diet contains less salt, phosphate, and protein.

People with kidney disease may have unfavorable effects from ingesting too much sodium because their kidneys cannot adequately eliminate additional sodium and fluid from the body. The buildup of sodium and fluid in the tissues and bloodstream can cause swelling in the legs, hands, and face, increased thirst, elevated blood pressure, heart failure, and shortness of breath.

Therefore, patients must keep an eye on and control their sodium consumption. Similar to hyperkalemia, excessive blood potassium levels can result in mortality, heart attacks, irregular heartbeats, slow heartbeats, and muscle weakness. Numerous foods contain phosphorus and potassium. As a result, patients with impaired kidney function should try to control their potassium and phosphorus levels. A renal diet puts a strong emphasis on getting enough high-quality protein while typically cutting back on fluid intake. Limiting potassium and calcium may also be necessary for some people. Because every person's body is unique, it is essential that every patient develop a diet that is suited to his or her individual requirements.

This book is a collection of renal-friendly recipes that will help you to create and consume a customized renal-friendly diet for a better life.

Chapter 1: Renal Diet Breakfast Recipes

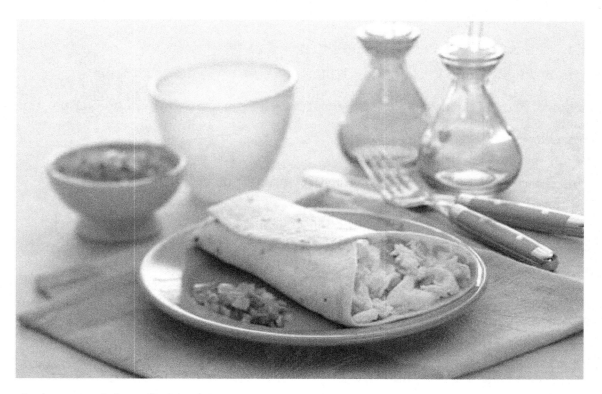

Here are the best renal-friendly breakfast recipes for people with compromised kidney function.

1. Loaded Veggie Eggs

Preparation time 5 mins Cooking Time 9 mins
Servings 2 persons
Nutritional facts 240 calories Carb 9 gm Protein 15 gm Fat 17 gm Sodium 194 mg Potassium 216 mg Phosphorous 165 mg
Ingredients

- Three cups of new spinach
- 1 minced garlic clove
- 4 whole eggs
- Black pepper, 1/4 teaspoon
- For garnish, use fresh parsley and spring onions.
- sliced 1/4 cup of onions
- Cauliflower, 1 cup
- 1 tablespoon of your preferred oil, such as coconut oil or avocado oil
- Bell peppers, cut into 1/4 cup

Instructions

- Eggs and pepper should be beaten till light and fluffy.
- Inside a big-sized griddle, warm the oil on moderate flame.
- Cook the peppers in the griddle with the onions till they are translucent as well as golden.
- Include cauliflower and spinach right away, then quickly whisk in the garlic.
- Sauté the vegetables for around 5 mins, then diminish the flame to moderate-low.
- Include the eggs and mix them into the veggies.

- Include fresh parsley or spring onions to the top of the eggs once they are fully cooked. If you don't need to limit your potassium intake, feel free to serve with a side of vibrant, fresh tomatoes sprinkled with coarse black pepper.

2. Egg and Sausage Breakfast Sandwich

Preparation time 3 mins Cooking Time 6 mins
Servings 1 person
Nutritional facts 253 calories Carb 26 gm Protein 17 gm Fat 9 gm Sodium 591 mg Potassium 218 mg
Phosphorous 158 mg
Ingredients

- 1 turkey sausage patty
- Quarter cup of liquid low-cholesterol egg substitute
- nonstick cooking spray
- 1 tablespoon of shredded natural sharp cheddar cheese
- 1 English muffin

Instructions

- Put the egg product into a small-sized griddle that has been sprayed using nonstick cooking spray, and cook across moderate flame. With a spoon, flip the egg when it seems almost done and cook for a further 30 secs.
- English muffin is toasted.
- The turkey sausage patty should be put on a dish, covered using a paper towel, & microwave for around one min or as directed on the package.
- Put a fried egg on an English muffin. Sharp cheddar cheese, Sausage patty, and the rest of the muffin half should be put on top.

3. 1-Min Breakfast: Quick and Easy Omelet

Preparation time 20 secs Cooking Time 40 secs
Servings 1 person
Nutritional facts 255 calories Carb 1.3 gm Protein 13 gm Fat 22 gm Sodium 145 mg Potassium 122 mg
Phosphorous 195 mg
Ingredients

- 1 TBSP. of butter (unsalted)
- Two eggs (comprising the yolk)
- Half cup of filling (vegetables, meat)
- Two tablespoons of water

Instructions

- Beat eggs with water.
- Warm the butter in a small-sized pot.
- Include the egg mixture to the pot.
- The mixture must quickly begin to solidify around the pot's edges.
- To allow the uncooked egg to fill the pot and cook, carefully push the cooked omelet parts from the outer borders toward the center using a spoon.
- Keep doing till the egg has set and stopped flowing.
- Include 1/2 cup of your chosen filling to one side of the omelet.
- Fold the omelet in half with the spoon to complete cooking.

4. Strawberry and Peanut Oatmeal Container

Preparation time 3 mins Cooking Time 2 mins
Servings 1 person
Nutritional facts 325 calories Carb 52 gm Protein 9 gm Fat 10 gm Sodium 164 mg Potassium 40 mg
Phosphorous 145 mg
Ingredients

- 1/2 cup of old fashioned oats
- two tbsps. unsalted peanuts
- one cup water
- half cup strawberries quartered
- one tbsp. maple syrup
- A quarter cup of plant-based milk optional
- 1/2 tsp. of cinnamon, optional

Instructions

- Put oats and water inside a serving container.
- Then put the container in oven for one and a half mins.
- Insert milk & maple syrup, if using.
- Mix well.
- Strawberries, peanuts, and cinnamon could be used for topping.

5. Avocado Toast

Preparation time 5 mins Cooking Time 5 mins
Servings 1 person
Nutritional facts 249 calories Carb 22 gm Protein 12 gm Fat 12 gm Sodium 313 mg Potassium 470 mg
Phosphorous 197 mg
Ingredients

- 1/4 avocado ripe
- 1 slice of whole grain bread
- 1 pinch of salt
- 1 tbsp. of balsamic drizzle
- quarter cup of grape tomatoes halved
- one egg
- quarter cup of arugula
- one pinch of black pepper

Instructions

- Bread should be toasted.
- Cook the egg the way you like.
- Avocado should be mashed over toast. Include salt & pepper as required.
- Include tomatoes, egg, and arugula to the avocado. It should also be sprinkled with balsamic.

6. Southwest Sweet Potato & Pineapple Hash

Preparation time five mins Cooking Time 15 mins
Servings 4 persons
Nutritional facts 246 calories Carb 5.2 gm Protein 9 gm Fat 14 gm Sodium 140 mg Potassium 593 mg
Phosphorous 149 mg
Ingredients

- one average onion sliced into half inch chunks
- one avocado
- one cup of pineapple sliced into 1/2" chunks
- 1 tbsp. of vegetable oil
- one red bell pepper sliced into half inch chunks
- 2 small-sized sweet potatoes peeled & sliced into 1/2" chunks
- A quarter tsp. of black pepper
- one teaspoon of ground cumin
- one tsp. of chili powder
- Four eggs over easy
- 1 lime
- 2 tsps. Of water

Instructions

- In a microwave-safe container, mix sweet potato with water. Wrap the dish in plastic wrap. Put in a microwave for around four mins till potatoes are cooked. Remove the plastic wrap and drain the potatoes (carefully – the steam is really hot). Using paper towels, dry.
- Warm the oil in a nonstick griddle over moderate-high flame. Mix the microwave potatoes, spices, bell pepper, onion, and one teaspoon of salt inside a mixing container. Cook for around 5 mins, or till peppers are tender, stirring occasionally.
- Whisk in the pineapple. Cook till pineapple is warmed, stirring regularly.
- Avocado should be mashed with the juice of half a lime. Insert 1 tsp. of salt. Cut the rest of the lime half into four wedges.
- It can be served with one cup of hash, 1 egg (boiled to your liking), 2 tablespoons mashed avocado, and a lime wedge.

7. Muffin Tin Eggs

Preparation time ten mins Cooking Time twenty mins
Servings twelve persons
Nutritional facts 345 calories Carb 11 gm Protein 9 gm Fat 8 gm Sodium 186 mg Potassium 413 mg Phosphorous 245 mg

Ingredients

- 3 oz. of cheese cheddar, shredded
- 1 tsp. of olive oil
- One and a half cups of packed spinach baby
- 4 tortillas as liked: gluten-free wrap, whole wheat, corn, etc.
- cooking spray
- 12 egg
- salt as required
- 3 tbsps. of milk lactose-free
- black pepper as required
- 12 tomato cherry, sliced
- A half cup of bell pepper diced

Instructions

- Warm up your oven at 350 ⁰ F.
- Warm up the pot on moderate-high flame. Sauté spinach in olive oil till wilted.
- In the meantime, whisk simultaneously the milk and eggs. Use salt & pepper as required.
- Slice twelve rounds out of your tortillas with a big biscuit cutter. Put tortillas in the wells of a twelve-well muffin tray that has been sprayed using cooking spray.

- Fill the wells with tomatoes, spinach, as well as bell pepper. After that, evenly distribute the egg mixture amongst the wells. Put cheddar cheese on top of every muffin.
- Bake the egg muffins for around 20 mins, or till puffed and set in the center.

8. Apple Fritter Donut

Preparation time eight mins Cooking Time 16 mins
Servings one person
Nutritional facts 145 calories Carb 15 gm Protein 1 gm Fat 9 gm Sodium 33 mg Potassium 67 mg Phosphorous 26 mg
Ingredients

- 1 cup of white flour (all-purpose)
- 4 big, tart cooking apples
- ⅓ cup of 1% low-fat milk
- Six tablespoons of sugar (divided use)
- 1 teaspoon of canola oil
- Three quarter cup of cooking oil for the frying
- 1 beaten big egg
- ⅓ cup of almond milk
- A half teaspoon of cinnamon
- one tsp. baking powder

Instructions

- Tart apples are to be peeled and cored.
- Every apple should be cut into 5 rings, every 1/2 inch thick.
- Sift simultaneously baking powder, flour, and 2 tablespoons of sugar into big-sized mixing dish.
- Mix almond milk, milk, egg, and 1 tsp. of oil inside a distinct container.
- Whisk the dry components with the milk and egg mixture and stir till barely mixed.
- Insert 1" cooking oil inside a deep griddle (around two-inches deep) after being heated at 375°F
- Dip the apple slices inside the fritter batter one at a time. Carefully put everyone in the hot oil inside the griddle and fry till golden brown (around 60-90 secs)
- Using paper towels, absorb excess oil.
- Mix the remainder of 1/4 cup sugar with the cinnamon & then sprinkle on top.
- Serve the apple fritter doughnuts while they're still warm.

9. Tasty Tuna Salad Sandwich

Preparation time ten mins Cooking Time, 0 mins
Servings 6 persons
Nutritional facts 178.96 calories Carb 3.56 gm Protein 22.15 gm Fat 6.53 gm Sodium 128.72 mg Potassium 218 mg Phosphorous 194 mg
Ingredients

- 18 oz. of Tuna, tinned in water, without salt, (3 oz.)
- 6 tbsps. of Sour cream
- 3 tsps. of Seasoned pepper, salt free
- A half cup of Celery, Sliced
- Salad dressing, mayonnaise type, regular, with the salt (cup)
- ¼ cup Onion, sliced
- 2 slices of the 45 Calories & Delightful, 100% Whole Wheat

Instructions

- All fresh vegetables should be thoroughly washed and dried prior to serving.
- Prior to using tinned tuna, drain it. Inside a moderate-sized mixing container, mix simultaneously all of the Ingredients and stir to mix. Allow for around one hr of refrigeration to allow flavors to mix.
- Serve right away or store inside the fridge for around three days.
- Preparing Sandwiches
- Follow the directions above to create the tuna salad spread.
- Portion between two slices of Sara Lee Delightful Wheat bread, spread 1/2 cup of salad. Serve right away.

10. Rava Uttapam: Gluten-Free, Low Potassium Recipe

Preparation time ten mins Cooking Time, 15 mins
Servings four persons
Nutritional facts 197 calories Carb 35 gm Protein 7 gm Fat 3 gm Sodium 245 mg Potassium 179 mg Phosphorous 169 mg
Ingredients

- Two tbsps. of Green Bell Pepper Finely Sliced, Capsicum
- 1 Cup of Rava or Semolina
- Two Green Chili
- .75 Cups of Water
- Two tbsps. of Red Bell Pepper Finely Sliced
- half Cup of Dahi, Yogurt
- Two tbsps. of Yellow Bell Pepper Finely Sliced
- Salt as required
- Two tsps. of Oil
- 1/2" Ginger

Instructions

- You have to dry roast 1 cup Rava or Semolina for 3 to 5 mins over moderate flame till it just becomes aromatic but does not change color.
- Put inside a container & put aside to cool.
- Include 1/2 cup dahi, salt, or Amchur for a low sodium, low potassium diet, and mix well after the Rava has cooled. Create certain there are no lumps.
- Include 1/2 cup water gradually and stir well to form a thick batter.
- Allow 10 to 15 mins for the batter to rest.
- Include 1/4 cup water just prior to you're ready to create Uttapam and stir well. A spoon should easily slide off the batter.
- Using a few drops of oil, grease an 8" non-stick pot.
- Warm the pot over moderate flame till it is hot.
- Diminish the flame to low and put 1/4 of the batter into the center of the pot (while your pot is still hot). Swirl the pot a little to help the batter spread.
- Sprinkle the bell pepper pieces on top and use a spoon to gently press them into the Uttapam. This will aid in the sticking of the bell pepper pieces to the uttapam.
- Flip the flame around moderate.
- Cook for two to three mins with the lid on.
- Remove the cover and gently loosen the Uttapam from the pot with a fliping spoon prior to flipping it over.
- Cook for a few mins more.

- Serve the hot Rava Uttapam with your favorite chutney.

11. Breakfast Quesadilla

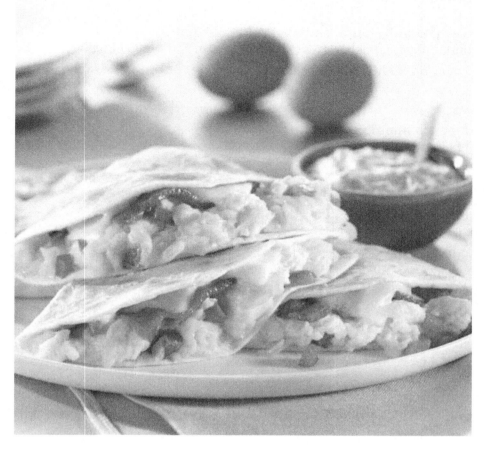

Preparation time 15 mins Cooking Time 16 mins
Servings 6 persons
Nutritional facts 160 calories Carb 8 gm Protein 14 gm Fat 10 gm Sodium 460 mg Potassium 135 mg
Phosphorous 260 mg
Ingredients

- Four eggs (beaten)
- One nonstick cooking spray
- Two 10-inch whole wheat flour tortillas
- Four slices of turkey bacon (cooked crisp & crumbled)
- One and a half cups of low-fat cheddar cheese, or use Monterey Jack, Mexican blend, or pepper jack(low-fat)
- tinned green chilies 1/4 cup
- A quarter tsp. of black pepper

Instructions

- Using cooking spray, mildly coat a small-sized griddle.
- Green chilies should be sautéed for one-two mins over moderate-low flame. Cook, stirring constantly, till the eggs are scrambled and set. Season using salt & pepper.
- Using frying spray, mildly coat a second, big-sized griddle. Put one tortilla in the griddle and cook on moderate flame for around one min, or till air bubbles appear. Cook for one min more on the other side (do not let tortilla get crispy).
- Half of the cheese should be spread evenly across the tortilla, all the way to the edges.

- Diminish the flame to a low setting. Put half of the cooked bacon as well as half of the egg mixture on top of the cheese. Cook for one min, or till the cheese begins to melt.
- To create a half-moon shape, fold the tortilla in half. Cook, flipping halfway through, till the folded tortilla is gently browned as well as the cheese filling is fully dissolved, around one to two mins.
- Put the quesadilla on a cutting board and put away. Rep with the second tortilla and the remainder cheese, bacon, as well as egg mixture in the griddle coated with frying spray.
- Slice every quesadilla into three wedges and serve with fresh salsa right away.

12. Kidney-Friendly Watermelon Power smoothie

Preparation time ten mins Cooking Time zero mins
Servings two persons
Nutritional facts 143 calories Carb 35.2 gm
Protein 4.1 gm Fat 0.9 gm Sodium41.1 mg Potassium887 mg Phosphorous 115 mg
Ingredients

- Two mint springs, leaves only
- 1 celery stalk
- Two cups of frozen watermelon
- 1 moderate cucumber, peeled & sliced
- Squeeze of lime

Instructions

- Cut the cucumber into slices after peeling it.
- Prepare the celery stalk by cutting it into squares and placing it inside the mixer.
- Inside a mixer, mix the frozen watermelon and cucumber. Mix the two mint springs leaves inside a container.
- Squeeze a lemon into your mixture.
- Blend till smooth and the desired smoothie texture has been achieved.
- It's time to drink.

13. Oven Turmeric Scrambled Eggs – Healthy Meal Prep

Preparation time 5 mins Cooking Time, 15 mins
Servings 5 persons
Nutritional facts 149 calories Carb 1.3 gm Protein 12.8 gm Fat 9.9 gm Sodium 192.4 mg Potassium 306.7 mg Phosphorous 297.8 mg
Ingredients

- half to one tsp. of turmeric powder
- Pinch of cumin (1/4 tsp. or so)
- 8 -10 big eggs
- Optional seasonings – Cilantro, avocado, cheese, salsa, etc.
- A half cup of almond milk, unsweetened or non-dairy milk
- 1/4 tsp. of black pepper & kosher salt every

Instructions

- Set your oven's temperature to 350 ⁰ F.
- Whisk the eggs, milk, turmeric, and other spices in a sizable mixing basin. Gently put the egg mixture into an oiled sheet pot.
- Bake the eggs for ten to twelve mins, or until they have started to set. A wooden spoon should be used to stir the eggs on the sheet pot prior to placing it back in the oven once the oven rack has been removed or carefully pulled out.

- Reflip the sheet pot to the oven for an include additional eight to ten mins, or until the scrambled eggs are almost set and the right consistency for you. Take one out of the oven, then mix another with a spoon.
- While still hot, garnish with Ingredients like cilantro and peppers. Alternately, store for around four days in an sealed container.
- Consequently, bake the eggs for 15 to 17 mins without scrambling them, then cut them into baked egg squares.
- Avocado, peppers, salsa, cilantro, and other veggies are available as extra seasonings.

14. Renal-Friendly Homemade Sausage Patties

Preparation time 13 mins Cooking Time, 22 mins
Servings 16 persons
Nutritional facts 173.3 calories Carb 0 gm Protein 9.8 gm Fat 14 gm Sodium 32.5 mg Potassium 65 mg Phosphorous 58 mg
Ingredients

- 1/8 tsp. of crushed red pepper flakes
- half cup of finely sliced onion
- one tablespoon of sugar or one tablespoon of brown sugar
- Two teaspoons of dried sage
- one pinch of ground cloves
- one tsp. of fresh thyme, finely sliced
- Two tablespoons of olive oil
- 1 big egg yolk
- One teaspoon of fresh ground black pepper
- Two lbs. of ground lean pork

Instructions

- Cook the onion in the olive oil over a low flame setting.
- Stir onions occasionally till they tenderen and brown.
- 8 to 10 mins
- Allow 10 mins for cooling.
- Mix the sage, red & black pepper, cloves, sugar, and thyme inside a small-sized container.
- Inside a big-sized mixing container, mix the pork, egg yolk, as well as reserved onion, then include the spices.
- Mix thoroughly.
- Create 16 patties, every weighing 2 ounces.
- Inside a big-sized griddle over moderate-high flame, pot-fry the patties for around five mins on every side or when the internal temperature reveryes 160 º F.

15. Turkey Sausage Patties with Apple

Preparation time ten mins Cooking Time, ten mins
Servings 12 persons
Nutritional facts 105 calories Carb 2 gm Protein 14 gm Fat 5 gm Sodium 260 mg Potassium 326 mg Phosphorous 198 mg
Ingredients

- A half tsp. of garlic powder
- A half tsp. of salt
- 1 lb. of 90-93% lean ground turkey
- A half tsp. of Italian seasoning or dried sage
- 1/4 tsp. of crushed fennel

- A half cup of finely minced apples
- A quarter tsp. of black pepper
- 1–2 Tbsp. of cooking fat of choice
- A half tsp. of paprika

Instructions

- Mix the turkey (or chicken), seasonings, salt, diced apple, and pepper in a mixing container. The components should be thoroughly mixed using a big spoon or your hands.
- Using damp hands, shape the meat mixture into twelve little patties.
- In a big griddle, heat the oil to a moderate-high flame. According to the size and non-stickiness of your pot, include a small amount of oil or fat to the heated griddle for every batch of patties, usually around 1/2 tablespoon.
- Arrange the patties in the pot, being careful not to crowd them or it will be difficult to flip them over and they won't brown as nicely. Cook until browned and the centre is no longer pink, around four to five mins on every side.
- Continue making patties with the rest of the oil and turkey mixture and put them on a platter covered with paper towels.
- Keep in the fridge in a covered container.

16-Greek Salad

Preparation time fifteen mins Cooking Time zero mins
Servings 3 persons
Nutritional facts 202 calories Carb 26 gm Protein 7 gm Fat 8 gm Sodium 97 mg Potassium 308 mg Phosphorous 267 mg
Ingredients

- Red pepper flakes, 1/4 teaspoon
- a one cup of sliced black pepper and red bell pepper
- Red wine vinegar, 1 tablespoon
- 1 can of garbanzo beans with little salt
- 0.5 tablespoons of lemon juice
- Dijon mustard, 1/4 teaspoon
- Olive oil, 1 tablespoon
- Don't use the stuffed green olives; instead, use 10 green olives per container.
- one cup of sliced cucumber
- sliced 1/4 cup red onion
- Garlic powder, 1/8 teaspoon

Instructions

- Slice the vegetables, comprising the olives, and put them inside a big-sized mixing container.
- Drain and wash the tinned garbanzo beans and include them to the container.
- Create the dressing and whisk the salad.

17. Maple Pancakes

Preparation time ten mins Cooking Time 20 mins
Servings twelve persons
Nutritional facts 178 calories Carb 25 gm Protein 6 gm Fat 6 gm Sodium 297 mg Potassium 126 mg Phosphorous 116 mg
Ingredients

- Canola oil, 2 tbsps.
- All-purpose flour, 1 cup
- maple extract, one tbsp.

- Baking powder, two tsps.
- Salt, 1/8 tsp.
- two substantial egg whites
- 1% low-fat milk, one cup
- one tbsp. of sugar, granulated

Instructions
- In a moderate mixing basin, mix the flour, salt, sugar, and baking powder. Create a well in the middle of the dry mixture. Take it out of the equation.
- In a sizable mixing basin, mix the egg whites, oil, milk, and maple extract.
- Include all of the egg mixture at once to the dry components. Only stir to moisten the mixture—the batter should still be lumpy.
- To create 4" pancakes, put around 1/4 cup of batter onto a hot, mildly greased heavy griddle or griddle.
- On a moderate temperature, cook for two mins on every end, or until golden brown. Flip the pancake when the top is bubbling and the edges are just beginning to dry out. To keep the pancakes airy and light, merely flip them once and avoid pressing with the spoon.

18. Healthier Lemon Muffins

Preparation time five mins Cooking Time 16 mins
Servings six persons
Nutritional facts 208 calories Carb 36 gm Protein 4 gm Fat 6 gm Sodium 257 mg Potassium 51 mg Phosphorous 98 mg
Ingredients
- 2 tbsps. of lemon juice, freshly squeezed
- One cup of white whole wheat flour, or all-purpose flour
- A half tsp. of baking powder
- A half tsp. of lemon juice, freshly squeezed
- A quarter tsp. of salt
- ¼ cup of maple syrup
- One big egg
- ⅓ cup of plain Greek yogurt
- Zest from one lemon
- A half cup of powdered sugar
- A half tsp. of almond milk/milk/cream
- ¼ cup of coconut oil, dissolved
- A half tsp. of vanilla extract
- One tsp. of vanilla extract
- A half tsp. of baking soda

Instructions
- Set the oven to 350 °F. Put away a muffin pot that has been coated with paper liners or sprayed with baking spray.
- The dissolved and cooled coconut oil, lemon juice, egg, Greek yoghurt, maple syrup, and vanilla extract should all be mixed in an average mixing container. To mingle, blend.
- Fill the mixing container with the baking soda, flour, salt, baking powder, and lemon zest. Just until mixed, stir.
- There should be enough batter to create six muffins, so fill the muffin tray 3/4 of the way full.
- Bake for approximately 16 mins, or until toothpick inserted in the center of the cake comes out clean.
- After taking it out of the oven, let it cool for around 5 mins prior to transferring it to a cooling rack to finish cooling.

- To create the icing, place all of the components in a small container and stir to mix. Douse the muffins in the glaze.

19. Best Classic Low Sodium Chili

Preparation time ten mins Cooking Time, 30 mins
Servings 18 persons
Nutritional facts 261 calories Carb 17.3 gm Protein 22.2 gm Fat 12 gm Sodium 94 mg Potassium 479 mg Phosphorous 171.2 mg
Ingredients

- 1 28-ounce can of crushed tomatoes without salt
- White sugar or dark brown sugar, 4 tablespoons
- 28-ounce can of salt-free fire-roasted tomatoes
- 4 teaspoons of ground cumin
- 3.5 cups of beef broth devoid of salt and water
- One 10-ounce can of green chilies and diced tomatoes without salt
- Garlic minced, three tablespoons
- 1 tablespoon of smoked paprika
- 90 percent lean ground beef or three pounds of quality meat Black pepper, ground, 1.5 teaspoons
- Olive oil, 3 tablespoons
- 3 fifteen.5-ounce cans of the unsalted kidney beans in red
- Chilli powder, 6 tablespoons
- 1 substantial green pepper
- 3 diced medium yellow onions
- ground cayenne pepper, 0.75 tsp.
- 6 tablespoons of tomato paste without any salt
- 2 teaspoons of cinnamon, toasted McCormick seasoning
- 1 fifteen-ounce can of sweet corn with no salt

Instructions

- Warm the olive oil in a big soup pot over a moderate-high temperature. Ground beef should be brown in a big pot. Prior to cutting it into smaller pieces, let it cook for a few mins. Cook for around six to seven mins, stirring now and then, or until the beef is mostly browned. Include the onion and green pepper to the meat when it is around 3/4 done, and whisk to mix.
- Include the broth or water and the rest of the tinned Ingredients. Everything should be properly mixed.
- In a mixing container, mix the garlic powder, chilli powder, cinnamon, pepper, cumin, sugar, smoked paprika, and optionally, cayenne pepper. Stir everything simultaneously thoroughly.
- The mixture should be brought to a gentle boil for around 5 mins. Flip down the heat to moderate-low, cover the pot, and gently simmer for 20 to 25 mins, stirring now and then.
- Stirring occasionally during the two hrs of simmering will help the flavour to fully develop and result in a much better chilli.
- In the kettle, extinguish the flame. Prior to serving, give the chilli 5 to 10 mins to rest.
- Prior to keeping in sealed containers in the fridge, allow it cool fully.

20. Chocolate Pancakes with Moon Pie Stuffing

Preparation time 11 mins Cooking Time twelve mins
Servings twelve persons

Nutritional facts 194 calories Carb 22 gm Protein 7 gm Fat 9 gm Sodium 121 mg Potassium 135 mg Phosphorous 134 mg

Ingredients

- Body Fortress vanilla whey protein powder, 2/3 cup
- Half a cup of creamed marshmallows
- 12 cup softened cream cheese
- Extract of vanilla, two tablespoons
- Brownie Pancakes
- Unsweetened cocoa powder in the amount of 3 teaspoons
- flour, 1 cup
- 1 cup of milk, 2%
- Baking soda, half a tsp.
- 1 egg
- Unsweetened cocoa powder, 1 tbsp
- Sugar, three tbsps.
- one-fourth cup of heavy cream
- Canola oil, 2 tbsps.
- Lemon juice, 1 tbsp.

Instructions

- In a mixing dish, mix the heavy cream and cocoa powder and whisk until stiff peaks form.
- Do not overmix. Whip the marshmallow cream, cream cheese, and whey protein powder for approximately a min, or until well blended. Put in the fridge with a cover.
- Mix all of the dry Ingredients in a sizable mixing basin and put away.
- Mix all of the wet Ingredients in a moderate-sized mixing container.
- Do not overmix; simply fold the wet and dry Ingredients simultaneously until they are mixed.
- Cooking pancakes on a moderate burner (375° F) with a mildly oiled griddle is recommended.
- Use around 1/8 cup batter to create 4-inch pancakes, flipping them as they start to bubble.

21. Fluffy Homemade Buttermilk Pancakes

Preparation time five mins Cooking Time, seven mins
Servings 9 persons
Nutritional facts 217 calories Carb 27 gm Protein 6 gm Fat 9 gm Sodium 330 mg Potassium 182 mg Phosphorous 100 mg

Ingredients

- Low-fat buttermilk in two cups
- Cream of tartar, 1 teaspoon
- two cups of regular flour
- Baking soda, 1 1/2 tablespoons
- two enormous eggs
- Canola oil (for cooking) in a quarter cup and a tbsp.
- Sugar, two tablespoons

Instructions

- Warm up a griddle over moderate-high flame.

- Inside a big-sized mixing container, mix simultaneously the dry components. Mix the dry Ingredients with the oil, buttermilk, and egg inside a mixing container. Blend the dry components with a whisk or a spoon till they are completely moist.
- Grease the griddle with a tablespoon of canola oil. Scoop the pancake batter onto the griddle with a 13-cup measuring cup. Every pancake should be around 4 inches in diameter. For easy flipping, leave around 2 inches between the pancakes. When the bubbles atop of the pancakes have mostly vanished, flip them with a spoon. Allow the other side to brown till it no longer appears wet in the center.
- Transfer to a serving dish.
- Consider serving with fresh berries as well as a side of eggs for a healthier twist.

22. Southwest Baked Egg Breakfast Cups

Preparation time 8 mins Cooking Time, 12 mins
Servings twelve persons
Nutritional facts 109 calories Carb 13 gm Protein 5 gm Fat 4 gm Sodium 79 mg Potassium 82 mg Phosphorous 91 mg
Ingredients
- Half tsp. black pepper
- Three cups rice, cooked
- two ounces of pimentos, drained and diced
- 4 ounces of green chilies, diced
- Half a teaspoon of ground cumin
- 2 eggs, beaten
- ½ cup of skim milk
- nonstick cooking spray
- Four ounces of cheddar cheese, shredded

Instructions
- In a sizable mixing container, mix the rice, 2 ounces of cheese, cumin, eggs, chilies, milk, pimentos, and pepper.
- muffin tins with nonstick cooking spray.
- Spread the mixture evenly into 12 muffin tins. Every cup should have the final two ounces of cheese strewn on top.
- Bake for 15 mins, or until the cheese is set, in a 400°F oven.

23. Spicy Tofu Scrambler

Preparation time 6 mins Cooking Time twenty mins
Servings two persons
Nutritional facts 213 calories Carb 10 gm Protein 18 gm Fat 13 gm Sodium 24 mg Potassium 467 mg Phosphorous 242 mg
Ingredients
- one cup firm tofu
- diced green bell pepper, 1/4 cup
- Garlic powder, 1/4 teaspoon
- 1/4 cup of red bell peppers, sliced
- onion powder, 1 teaspoon
- 1 minced garlic clove
- one-eighth tsp. of turmeric
- Olive oil, one tsp.

Instructions

- You have to sauté garlic as well as both the bell peppers inside olive oil and in a moderate-sized nonstick griddle.
- Tofu should be washed and drained prior to crumbling it inside the griddle. Mix the rest of the Ingredients and stir well.
- Cook, stirring occasionally, till tofu becomes light brown, approximately 20 mins. The water in the mixture will evaporate.
- Warm tofu scrambler should be served.

24. Blueberry Muffins

Preparation time ten mins Cooking Time thirty mins
Servings twelve persons
Nutritional facts 275 calories Carb 44 gm Protein 5 gm Fat 9 gm Sodium 210 mg Potassium 121 mg Phosphorous 100 mg
Ingredients

- two cups of regular flour
- Unsalted butter, half a cup
- 2 cups of milk, 1%
- Sugar, two teaspoons (for topping)
- 1 1/4 cups sugar
- Baking powder, two teaspoons
- 2 eggs
- 1/2 tsp. of salt
- 2 1/2 cups of blueberries, fresh

Instructions

- Blend the sugar and margarine in a mixer set at low-speed till creamy and fluffy.
- Mix inside the eggs one at a time till well mixed.
- Sift the dry Ingredients and include the milk.
- You have to mash half cup blueberries. Then mix in the rest of the blueberries.
- Vegetable oil should be sprayed into the muffin cups and on the pot's surface. In a muffin tin, put muffin cups.
- Fill every muffin around the brim with muffin mixture. Sugar should be sprinkled on the tops of the muffins.
- Warm up your oven at 375°F and bake for 25–30 mins. Allow to cool for around 30 min in the pot prior to carefully removing.

25. Dilly Scrambled Eggs

Preparation time three mins Cooking Time, 7 mins
Servings one person
Nutritional facts 194 calories Carb 1 gm Protein 16 gm Fat 14 gm Sodium 213 mg Potassium 192 mg Phosphorous 250 mg
Ingredients

- 1 teaspoon of dried dill weed
- Two big eggs
- One tablespoon of crumbled goat cheese
- 1/8 tsp. of black pepper

Instructions

- Inside a mixing container, whisk the eggs and then put them into a nonstick griddle over moderate flame.
- Whisk eggs with dill weed and black pepper.
- Cook till the eggs have become scrambled.
- Prior to serving, top with crumbled goat cheese.

26. Great Way to Start Your Day Bagel

Preparation time 3 mins Cooking Time four mins
Servings four persons
Nutritional facts 134 calories Carb 19 gm Protein 5 gm Fat 6 gm Sodium 219 mg Potassium 162 mg Phosphorous 50 mg
Ingredients
- Two red onion slices
- One bagel, 2 ounces' size
- Two tablespoons of cream cheese
- 1 teaspoon of low-sodium lemon pepper seasoning
- 2 tomato slices, around 1/4-inch thick
Instructions
- Bagel should be sliced and toasted till golden brown.
- Cream cheese should be spread over every bagel half. The tomato slice and onion slice should be put on top and sprinkled using lemon pepper.

27. Apple and oat cereal

Preparation time three mins Cooking Time, three mins
Servings one person
Nutritional facts 248 calories Carb 33 gm Protein 11 gm Fat 8 gm Sodium 164 mg Potassium 362 mg Phosphorous 240 mg
Ingredients
- One big egg
- 1/3 cup of quick-cooking oatmeal
- Half moderate apple
- 1/4 teaspoon of cinnamon
- Half cup of almond milk
Instructions
- A half apple should be cored and finely sliced
- In a big-sized mug, mix the egg, oats, and almond milk. With a fork, thoroughly mix the Ingredients. Whisk in the apple and cinnamon. Stir once more till everything is well mixed.
- Cook for around two mins on high in the microwave. Using a fork, fluff the mixture. If necessary, cook for another 30 to 60 secs.
- If you want a thinner cereal, include a little more milk or water.

28. Egg n Milk

Preparation time three mins Cooking Time three mins
Servings one person
Nutritional facts 117 calories Carb 3 gm Protein 15 gm Fat 5 gm
Sodium 194 mg Potassium 226 mg Phosphorous 138 mg
Ingredients
- Two tablespoons of 1% low fat milk
- One big egg
- 1/8 tsp. of black pepper

- two big egg whites

Instructions

- Using cooking spray, coat a 12-ounce coffee cup. In a mug, whisk simultaneously the milk, egg, & egg whites till smooth.
- Cook for 45 secs in a microwave-safe coffee cup; remove and stir. Microwave for another 30-45 secs, or till the eggs are nearly set.
- Enjoy with a pinch of black pepper.

29. Yummy Omelet

Preparation time 4 mins Cooking Time ten mins
Servings 1 person
Nutritional facts 255 calories Carb 1.3 gm Protein 13 gm Fat 28 gm Sodium 145 mg Potassium 122 mg Phosphorous 195 mg

Ingredients

- 1 tablespoon of unsalted butter
- 2 eggs
- A half cup of filling (meat, vegetables, seafood)
- Two tablespoons of water

Instructions

- In a mixing dish, include the eggs and water, and whisk to mix.
- Butter should sizzle when heated in a ten-inch omelet griddle or fry pot.
- In the pot, put the egg mixture. The mixture's edges ought to start to set right away. Using an inverted pancake flipper, gently push cooked sections towards the centre so that uncooked portions can touch the hot pot surface. When necessary, tilt and adjust the pot.
- As long as the egg is still oozing, keep going. You can fill the omelet with half a cup of veggies, meat, or shellfish if you choose. Put the filling on the left side if you are a right-handed person and the right side if you are a left-handed person.
- Using the pancake flipper, fold the omelet in half. The lower part of the omelet should be facing up as you invert it onto a plate.

30. Anytime Energy Bars

Preparation time 7 mins Cooking Time 40 mins
Servings eight persons
Nutritional facts 206 calories Carb 27 gm Protein 7 gm Fat 45 gm Sodium 35 mg Potassium 182 mg Phosphorous 163 mg

Ingredients

- 3 tbsps. of sliced, unsalted peanuts
- Rolling oats in a cup
- applesauce, 1/3 cup
- Semi-sweet tiny chocolate chips amounting to 1/4 cup
- 1/3 cup of coconut shavings
- Three big eggs
- Honey, 3 tablespoons
- 1/8 tsp. of cinnamon powder

Instructions

- Warm up your oven at 325 ⁰ F. Spray a nine-by-nine-inch baking pot using cooking spray.
- Mix peanuts, oats, chocolate chips, cinnamon, and coconut inside a big-sized mixing container.
- Inside a small-sized mixing container, whisk simultaneously the eggs. Mix in the honey and applesauce thoroughly.

- Mix the egg mixture into the oat mixture thoroughly.
- In a greased 9x9 pot, press the mixture evenly into the lower part.
- Cooking Time, is 40 mins. Allow to cool prior to cutting into bars.
- Keep refrigerated for around one week in a sealed bowl.

31. Apple Bran Muffins

Preparation time 8 mins Cooking Time twenty-five mins
Servings twelve persons
Nutritional facts 234 calories Carb 40 gm Protein 7 gm Fat 26 gm Sodium 287 mg Potassium 446 mg Phosphorous 121 mg
Ingredients

- a half-cup of raisins
- two cups whole wheat flour,
- one and a half cups wheat bran
- 1 orange's juice
- Baking soda, 1 1/4 teaspoons
- one tbsp. of grated orange rind
- one cup of apple pieces
- sliced nuts or sunflower seeds equaling 1/2 cup
- one and a quarter tablespoons of baking soda
- scant 2 cups of sour milk or buttermilk
- Nutmeg, half a teaspoon
- one and a half cups of wheat bran
- Oil, two tbsps.
- Nutmeg, half a tsp.

Instructions

- Warm up your oven at 350 ° F.
- Combine simultaneously baking soda, flour, bran, and nutmeg with a fork.
- Mix the raisins, apples, orange rind, as well as nuts or seeds inside a mixing container.
- To create 2 cups, put 1 orange's juice into a 2 cup measure as well as include buttermilk.
- Stir simultaneously the buttermilk, molasses, egg, and oil till thoroughly mixed.
- With a few quick strokes, mix liquid and dry Ingredients.
- Fill muffin tins two-thirds full with batter and bake for twenty-five mins.

32. Apple Filled Crepes

Preparation time 6 mins Cooking Time eight mins
Servings one person
Nutritional facts 315 calories Carb 40 gm Protein 5 gm Fat 52.5 gm Sodium 356 mg Potassium 160 mg Phosphorous 103 mg
Ingredients

- flour, one cup
- four egg yolks
- a half-cup of sugar
- two glasses of milk

- Cinnamon, half a tsp.
- four apple
- Brown sugar, half a cup
- oil, 1/4 cup
- 2 whole eggs
- 1/2 cup or one stick of unsalted butter
- Nutmeg, half a teaspoon

Instructions

- Mix the oil, egg yolks, flour, whole eggs, sugar, and milk inside a mixing container till the batter is smooth and lump-free.
- Over moderate flame, warm a small-sized nonstick griddle.
- Coat the pot using cooking spray.
- Use a 2-ounce ladle or a 1/4 cup, spoon 1 scoop of batter into the pot at this point. The pancake batter will now be finely spread throughout the pot's lower part as you swirl the pot.
- With the use of a rubber spoon, fry the pancake for around 30 secs prior to flipping it over and cooking for an additional 10 secs. Crepes should be left aside while the filling is being prepared. Apples should be peeled, cored, and sliced into 12 slices every.
- Warm a moderate sauté pot.
- Brown sugar is included after the butter has dissolved.
- Mix the cinnamon, apples, and nutmeg inside a mixing container.
- Cook till the apples are tender but not mushy. Allow to cool prior to serving.
- Fill around two tablespoons of apple stuffing into the middle of every crepe.
- Then it should be rolled into a log.

33. Banana Oat Shake

Preparation time 7 mins Cooking Time zero mins
Servings two persons
Nutritional facts 172 calories Carb 33 gm Protein 6 gm Fat 19.7 gm Sodium 42 mg Potassium 297 mg
Phosphorous 160 mg
Ingredients

- Amount of vanilla extract: one and a half tsps.
- Muesli boiled in half cup, cold
- skim milk, two-third cup
- Brown sugar, two tbsps.
- A serving of wheat germ
- Banana, half frozen, sliced into pieces

Instructions

- The oatmeal should be put inside mixer and blended for a few mins.
- Then wheat germ, milk, vanilla, brown sugar, and half banana should be included. Then it should be blended till thick and smooth.

34. Banana-Apple Smoothie

Preparation time 4 mins Cooking Time, zero mins
Servings one person
Nutritional facts 292 calories Carb 61 gm Protein 9 gm Fat 24 gm Sodium 103 mg Potassium 609 mg
Phosphorous 140 mg
Ingredients

- One tablespoon of honey
- 1/2 banana, peeled & cut into chunks
- Quarter cup of skim milk
- half cup unsweetened applesauce
- Half cup plain yogurt
- 2 tablespoons of oat bran

Instructions
- Put yogurt, applesauce, milk, banana, and honey inside mixer.
- All the Ingredients should be blended till smooth.

35. Berrylicious Smoothie

Preparation time 3 mins Cooking Time, 0 mins
Servings two persons
Nutritional facts 115 calories Carb 18 gm Protein 6 gm Fat 3 gm Sodium 14 mg Potassium 223 mg Phosphorous 80 mg
Ingredients
- 1/2 cup of blueberries, frozen & unsweetened
- Quarter cup of cranberry juice cocktail
- one tsp. of vanilla extract
- two-third cup of silken tofu, firm
- Half cup of raspberries, frozen & unsweetened
- A half a teaspoon of powdered lemonade, such as Country Time
- 2/3 cup of silken tofu, firm

Instructions
- Juice should be put into a mixer.
- The rest of the Ingredients should be included next.
- Blend till very smooth.
- Should be served immediately.

36. Biscuits with Master Mix

Preparation time 3 mins Cooking Time, seventeen mins
Servings twelve persons
Nutritional facts 174 calories Carb 18 gm Protein 3 gm Fat 10 gm Sodium 171 mg Potassium 81 mg Phosphorous 51 mg
Ingredients
- Two third cup of Water
- Three cups of Master Mix

Instructions
- Warm up your oven at 450 º F (230 º Celsius).
- Blend all of the Ingredients thoroughly.
- Allow 5 mins for cooling.
- Knead dough 15 times on a mildly floured surface.
- Roll out to a thickness of half inch and slice with a flour cutter into 12 biscuits.
- On an ungreased baking sheet, put 2 inches apart.
- Warm up your oven at 350°F and bake for ten-twelve mins, or till golden brown.

37. Blueberry Squares

Preparation time 6 mins Cooking Time sixty mins
Servings sixteen persons

Nutritional facts 247 calories Carb 40 gm Protein 2 gm Fat 18 gm Sodium 3 mg Potassium 38 mg Phosphorous 17 mg

Ingredients

- Cinnamon, one tsp.
- Sugar, 3/4 cup
- One sugar cup
- 3 cups of berries, blue
- flour, one and a half cups
- Oats in a cup
- zest from one lemon
- one and a half sticks or three-quarter cup of dissolved butter
- water, 1 cup
- corn flour, 3 tablespoons

Instructions

- Warm up your oven at 350 °F (180 °C).
- Mix cinnamon, flour, sugar, oats, and butter simultaneously inside a moderate mixing container till crumbly.
- In a 9-inch square pot, press half of the flour-oat mixture.
- Cover the lower part of the pot with lemon zest and blueberries.
- Inside a microwave-safe container, mix sugar and cornstarch, then slowly stir in water till just boiling.
- Over the blueberries, put the water, cornstarch, and sugar mixture.
- Over the top, sprinkle the rest of the flour/oat mixture.
- Allow 45 mins to 1 hr for cooking.

38. Bran Breakfast Bars

Preparation time 21 mins Cooking Time, 24 mins
Servings 12 persons
Nutritional facts 158 calories Carb 24 gm Protein 4 gm Fat 24 gm Sodium 2 mg Potassium 148 mg Phosphorous 142 mg

Ingredients

- One and a half cups of pure bran
- 1 cup of boiling water
- 1/3 cup of oil (soybean, corn, or safflower)
- 1/2 cup of whole wheat flour
- 1/3 cup of sliced raisins or med. dates, diced
- 3 tablespoons of brown-type granular sugar substitute
- 1 cup of oatmeal

Instructions

- Put the fruit that has been diced in a dish of boiling water.
- Allow it to settle for around 20 mins.
- All the dry Ingredients should be mixed in a sizable mixing dish.
- Include boiling water to the liquid left over after draining the fruit to create 1 cup of liquid. Then include the oil and put it into the mixer, and process for around a min.
- Put immediately into the dry Ingredients and carefully mix.
- After comprising the fruit, re-mix.
- Put the batter into an 8" x 10" nonstick baking dish.

- Cuttings should be marked in 6 rows long and 4 rows narrow, levelling every row with your fingertips or a spoon in between.
- Cook in a warmed up oven for 22 mins at 375°F.
- Put there to cool on a wire rack.
- It should be chilled or frozen if you intend to preserve it for more than two days.

39. Burritos Rapidos

Preparation time 3 mins Cooking Time, ten mins
Servings 4 persons
Nutritional facts 232 calories Carb 16 gm Protein 14 gm Fat 80 gm Sodium 152 mg Potassium 211 mg Phosphorous 207 mg
Ingredients
- Eight beaten eggs
- One and a half teaspoons of canola or olive oil
- 4 corn tortillas (6-inch)
- Four green onions (scallions), cut fine
- half red bell pepper, diced

Instructions
- Warm the oil in a moderate frying pot across a moderate temperature.
- Cook for around three mins, or until green onion and bell pepper are tender.
- The eggs should be scrambled for around 5 mins, or until completely done.
- Put the tortillas between two wet paper towels on a platter.
- Microwave tortillas that have been toasted for two mins.
- The egg mixture should be put inside warm tortillas.
- Delight in the tortillas.

40. Fresh Fruit Lassi

Preparation time 4 mins Cooking Time, zero mins
Servings 2 persons
Nutritional facts 169 calories Carb 29 gm Protein 9 gm Fat 14 gm Sodium 143 mg Potassium 98 mg Phosphorous 59 mg
Ingredients
- Cardamom, 1/4 teaspoon, optional
- 1 cup of unflavored yoghurt
- Rose water, 1/2 tsp. (optional)
- 1/2 cup mango juice, peach nectar, or apricot nectar
- Lime juice, 1/4 cup (optional)
- a half-cup of milk
- As required, include 1-3 teaspoons of sugar.

Instructions
- Insert all components into mixer.
- Next, mix for two mins.
- Now put into distinct glasses and serve.

41. Fruit Bars

Preparation time 7 mins Cooking Time thirty mins
Servings twenty-four persons
Nutritional facts 131 calories Carb 21 gm Protein 1 gm Fat 17 gm Sodium 24 mg Potassium 14 mg Phosphorous 120 mg
Ingredients

- Vanilla extract, one tsp.
- two cups flour.
- Strawberry, raspberry, grape, and blackberry jam, one cup
- water, quarter cup
- one egg
- a half-cup of sugar
- Baking powder, one tsp.
- Vegetable oil, half a cup

Instructions

- Set your oven's temperature to 400°.
- In a mixing dish, mix sugar, flour, and baking powder.
- until it is crumbly, include the oil and stir.
- Thoroughly incorporate the water, egg, and vanilla essence.
- A greased 9x9 or 8x8 inch pot should be pushed with two thirds of the batter.
- The jam should be dispersed equally.
- The excess batter can be used to create topping crumbs.
- Bake for 25–30 mins after warming up the oven to 350°F.
- Prior to slicing into 24 bars, let it cool in the pot.

42. Fruit Julius

Preparation time 4 mins Cooking Time zero mins
Servings four persons
Nutritional facts 87 calories Carb 9 gm Protein 7 gm Fat 7 gm Sodium 108 mg Potassium 209 mg
Phosphorous 73 mg
Ingredients

- 3 ice cubes, crushed
- Half cup of juice: cranberry, orange, grape or other
- 2 teaspoons of tang powder
- Half cup of egg substitute

Instructions

- Mix all Ingredients with the exception of ice till smooth.
- Include ice.
- Blend till slushy.

43. Katie Shake

Preparation time three mins Cooking Time zero mins
Servings one person
Nutritional facts 144 calories Carb 21 gm Protein 5 gm Fat 12 gm Sodium 97 mg Potassium 209 mg
Phosphorous 137 mg
Ingredients

- A quarter prepared Jell-O
- 1/4 cup of plain yogurt or cottage cheese
- A quarter cup of vanilla ice cream

Instructions

- Mix the entire components inside mixer.
- Mix till smooth.

44. Lemon Apple Honey Smoothie

Preparation time 3 mins Cooking Time, zero mins
Servings four persons
Nutritional facts 170 calories Carb 38 gm Protein 2 gm Fat 7 gm Sodium 37 mg Potassium 327 mg
Phosphorous 59 mg
Ingredients

- Two to three teaspoons of honey
- A quarter cup of lemon juice
- 1 apple, peeled & cored
- 1/2 cup of apple juice
- One banana
- 1 cup of vanilla yogurt, frozen

Instructions

- Mix all of the Ingredients inside a mixer.
- Mix till smooth.

45. Lemon-Blueberry Corn Muffins

Preparation time 6 mins Cooking Time twenty mins
Servings twelve persons
Nutritional facts 117 calories Carb 19 gm Protein 3 gm Fat 2 gm Sodium 76 mg Potassium 92 mg
Phosphorous 71 mg
Ingredients

- Two tablespoons of lemon juice
- 3/4 cup of whole wheat flour
- One and a half teaspoons of the baking powder
- 1/4 cup of granulated sugar
- Three quarter cup of yellow cornmeal
- 1 beaten egg
- Two tablespoons of oil or unsalted butter, dissolved
- One teaspoon of lemon zest
- Three quarter cup of milk (cow's, rice, or soy)
- 1 cup of frozen or fresh blueberries

Instructions

- Increase the temperature of your oven to 400 º. Use nonstick cooking spray to coat a muffin tray or an 8-inch baking pot.
- In a big mixing container, mix cornmeal, baking powder, flour, and sugar.
- In a small container, mix the milk, oil or butter, lemon juice, egg, and lemon zest.
- Simply whisk the milk mixture into the cornmeal mixture. It's acceptable if there are some lumps.
- The blueberries are then gently incorporated into the mixture.
- Put the batter into a square or muffin pot that is 8 inches in size.
- for using an 8x8 pot, bake for 25 mins as opposed to 15 mins for preparing muffins.
- If desired, put some honey on top.

46-Maple Sausage

Preparation time 24 hrs Cooking Time, ten mins
Servings 12 persons
Nutritional facts 152 calories Carb 1 gm Protein 13 gm Fat 45 gm Sodium 43 mg Potassium 183 mg
Phosphorous 129 mg

Ingredients
- half pound of turkey meat
- one pound of meat or pork ground up
- Maple syrup, two tbsps.
- Black pepper, half a tsp.
- water, one tsp.
- 1/fourth of a tsp. of ground spices
- 2 tbsps. of fresh sage or 3/4 tsp. of dried sage
- 1/8 tsp. of nutmeg or mace

Instructions
- Take a big-sized container and combine the entire components.
- It should be refrigerated for around four hrs, or overnight.
- Create patties.
- Next, cook in griddle over moderate-high flame till well browned for around ten mins.

47. Master Mix

Preparation time 12 mins Cooking Time zero mins
Servings 13 persons
Nutritional facts 640 calories Carb 67 gm Protein 11 gm Fat 15 gm Sodium 164 mg Potassium 40 mg Phosphorous 145 mg
Ingredients
- two tsps. of cream of tartar
- Eight half cups of all-purpose flour
- One and a half cups of instant nonfat milk powder
- 1 tablespoon of baking powder
- Two quarter cups of vegetable shortening
- 1 teaspoon of baking soda

Instructions
- Mix the baking soda, milk powder, cream of tartar, flour, and baking powder.
- Using a pastry mixer, incorporate the shortening into the mixture until it is distributed evenly.
- Keep in a big, sealed bowl in a cold, dry location.
- You should be able to use it in 10–12 weeks.

48. Mexican Brunch Eggs

Preparation time 3 mins Cooking Time, 2 mins
Servings eight persons
Nutritional facts 214 calories Carb 13 gm Protein 9 gm Fat 10 gm Sodium 147 mg Potassium 240 mg Phosphorous 91 mg
Ingredients
- 2 smashed garlic cloves
- 1/2 cup of onion, sliced
- 8 toasty pieces of bread
- 1 1/2 tbsps. of cumin powder
- one eighth of a tsp. of cayenne
- 2 tbsps. of butter
- 8 beaten eggs
- one and a half cups thawed frozen corn,

Instructions
- In a big-sized griddle, sauté onion, margarine and garlic till onion is tender.
- Stir in the cumin, corn, and cayenne pepper.

- Put in the eggs or egg substitute & cook, occasionally stirring, on low flame till the eggs are set.
- On a big-sized platter, arrange toast triangles.
- Using a spoon spread the egg mixture on the toast triangles.
- Serve right away.

49. Pumpkin Spiced Applesauce Bread or Muffins

Preparation time 18 mins Cooking Time one hr twenty mins
Servings 12 persons
Nutritional facts 252 calories Carb 38 gm Protein 3 gm Fat 18 gm Sodium 141 mg Potassium 82 mg Phosphorous 41 mg
Ingredients

- Brown sugar, 1 cup
- Applesauce, unsweetened, in a cup and a half
- 2 eggs
- Baking soda, 1 teaspoon
- Baking powder, half a teaspoon
- Pumpkin pie spice, 2 teaspoons
- Vegetable oil, half a cup
- two cups of regular flour

Instructions

- Set your oven's temperature to 350 ⁰ F.
- Apply cooking spray to a loaf pot or muffin tin to grease.
- In a moderate mixing container, mix eggs, oil, brown sugar, and applesauce.
- The rest of the components should be mixed in a moderate-sized mixing basin.
- Just mix the flour mixture and applesauce mixture by stirring.
- To create a loaf or muffins, put the batter into the pot.
- If creating a loaf, bake for fifty to sixty mins.
- Approximately 20 mins should be spent baking muffins.
- To check if it's finished, poke it with a toothpick; it should come out clean.

50. Tropical Fruit Salad with Basil Lime Syrup

Preparation time five mins Cooking Time, 8 mins
Servings 10 persons
Nutritional facts 69 calories Carb 18 gm Protein 2 gm Fat 2 gm Sodium 0 mg Potassium 160 mg Phosphorous 16 mg
Ingredients

- one-fourth cup of water
- one and a half cups of sliced strawberries;
- one and a half tbsps. of lime zest.
- 2 cups of pineapple dice.
- A banana slice in three-quarter cup
- Sugar, quarter cup
- one cup of mango dice
- a container with quarter cup of basil leaves

Instructions

- In a small saucepot, bring the water to a boil and include the sugar.
- It must be brought to a boil until the sugar dissolves.
- Mix in the basil and lime zest after taking the pot from the heat.
- While the syrup cools, mix the fruit in a sizable mixing dish.

- Remove the sediments from the syrup by straining it through cheesecloth or a strainer.
- Include some fruit, then indulge.

51. Tutti-Frutti Mocha Mix Muffins

Preparation time 12 mins Cooking Time, 35 mins
Servings twelve persons
Nutritional facts 195 calories Carb tbd Protein 3 gm Fat 10 gm Sodium 129 mg Potassium 6 mg Phosphorous 74 mg
Ingredients

- one hen
- Mocha Mix, 3/4 cup
- One fruit cocktail 8-ounce can
- 1/3 cup of brown sugar
- two cups of flour.
- Ground allspice, one teaspoon
- Vegetable oil, 1/4 cup
- Baking powder, one tablespoon

Instructions

- Set your oven's temperature to 400 °F.
- Completely drain the fruit cocktail in a sieve.
- Sift the flour, baking powder, and allspice simultaneously, then set it aside.
- The oil, egg, and Mocha Mix should be whisked simultaneously in that sequence in a moderate-sized mixing dish.
- Now is the time to include the brown sugar.
- All of the dry Ingredients should be mixed at once and moistened.
- The consistency of the batter should be lumpy.
- To create 12 two and a half inch muffins, fold the fruit into the batter and put the mixture into paper baking cups.
- Bake for twenty-five mins, or until golden brown and firm to the touch, in a 350°F oven.
- Serve right away after removing from the pot.

52. Savory Crustless Quiche

Preparation time 3 mins Cooking Time, two mins
Servings four persons
Nutritional facts 195.5 calories Carb 21.7 gm Protein 11.4 gm Fat 7.2 gm Sodium 174.6 mg Potassium 344.8 mg Phosphorous 193.25 mg
Ingredients

- optional teaspoon of salt, pepper, or other spices,
- half cup of flour
- Three big eggs
- 1 cup of milk, 2%
- 1 cup of sliced onions
- 2/3 cup of tinned, unsalted green beans
- 1 cup of sliced mushrooms
- three diced bacon pieces

Instructions

- Crack the eggs into a mixing dish and whisk in every component, dairy first, then flour, until most lumps are gone. Put the spices, salt, and pepper in if using.
- Cook the filling Ingredients in a griddle over moderate heat for 15-20 mins, or until well cooked and bubbling.

- A deep-dish pie plate or an 8-inch cake pot should be generously sprayed with cooking spray because the quiche will stick if it isn't. Cooked filling should be put halfway into a greased baking pot, then tenderly spread to distribute evenly. Bake at 350 º F for forty to forty-five mins, or until the top is golden brown and a knife inserted in the center comes out clean.

53. Nutritious Burritos

Preparation time three mins Cooking Time five mins
Servings two persons
Nutritional facts 257 calories Carb 20 gm Protein 15 gm Fat 12 gm Sodium 384 mg Potassium 246 mg Phosphorous 184 mg
Ingredients

- Salsa, 2 tablespoons
- 1/4 teaspoon of cumin powder
- frying-pot nonstick coating
- 4 eggs
- 1/2 tsp. spicy pepper sauce
- 3 teaspoons of diced green chilli
- 2 burrito-sized flour tortillas

Instructions

- Spray nonstick cooking spray in a moderate-sized griddle and heat it over moderate heat.
- Mix eggs, cumin, green chilies, and hot sauce in a mixing container.
- Then include the eggs into the griddle and heat for one to two mins, or until done, while continually stirring.
- The next step is to reheat the tortillas, either in a separate griddle across moderate flame or in the microwave for twenty secs.
- Every tortilla needs to have half of the egg mixture on it prior to being wrapped up burrito-style.
- Every tortilla should be served with one tablespoon of salsa.

54. Spinach Ricotta Frittata

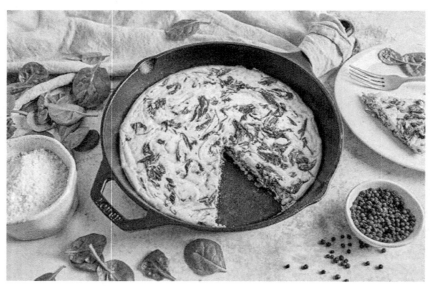

Preparation time 7 mins Cooking Time fifteen mins
Servings 6 persons
Nutritional facts 220 calories Carb 6 gm Protein 16 gm Fat 15 gm Sodium 164 mg Potassium 40 mg Phosphorous 145 mg
Ingredients

- 10 Omega 3 eggs

- 1 tablespoon of minced fresh herbs
- 1 minced garlic clove
- Olive oil, 1 tablespoon
- Ricotta cheese, 1 cup
- 2 cups of uncooked spinach
- 1 moderate onion, sliced

Instructions

- Set your oven's temperature to 350 º F.
- Olive oil should be used to sauté the garlic and onion in a nonstick, oven-safe pot.
- Cook the spinach after including it until it wilts.
- In a mixing container, mix the ricotta cheese, eggs, and fresh herbs.
- Include the egg mixture to the pot.
- Finish cooking the frittata in the oven for around 10 mins, or until the top has completely set.

55. Mushroom and Leek Pie

Preparation time 10 mins Cooking Time 30 mins
Servings 2 persons
Nutritional facts 184 calories Carb 11 gm Protein 8 gm Fat 12 gm Sodium 166 mg Potassium 122 mg
Phosphorous 101 mg
Ingredients

- mushrooms, diced into a half cup.
- 9-inch prepared pastry shell
- Olive oil, 1 tablespoon
- Grated parmesan cheese, two tablespoons
- pepper, black
- based on the depth of the shell, 8–10 eggs
- new thyme
- Leeks, cut into a half-cup

Instructions

- Set your oven's temperature to 350 º F.
- Leeks should be properly washed to remove any sand.
- Sauté leeks and mushrooms in one tablespoon of olive oil.
- Then season with fresh thyme and black pepper.
- Sautéed leeks and mushrooms should be dispersed throughout the pastry shell's base.
- Put the beaten eggs and cheese over the leeks and mushrooms in the pastry shell.
- Bake for 30 mins or until the mixture is set.

56. Blueberry Pancakes

Preparation time 6 mins Cooking Time eight mins
Servings one person
Nutritional facts 223 calories Carb 35 gm Protein 7 gm Fat 6 gm Sodium 196 mg Potassium 128 mg
Phosphorous 100 mg
Ingredients

- Sugar, 3 tablespoons
- 1.5 cups of simple all-purpose flour, sifted
- Dissolved two tablespoons of unsalted margarine

- 1 cup of frozen blueberries, thawed, or 1 cup of blueberries in a can, washed
- 2 mildly beaten eggs
- Buttermilk, 1 cup
- Baking powder, two teaspoons

Instructions

- Sift the flour, sugar, and baking powder into a mixing container.
- Create a well in the centre and fill it with the rest of the Ingredients.
- Start at the centre and include the dry Ingredients gradually to create a smooth batter. Cooking should begin immediately.
- Warm up a 12-inch heavy griddle or griddle with a little oil.
- Using a 1/3 cup measuring cup, portion out the pancakes and cook them until done, simply flipping once.

57. Bannock (Lusknikn)

Preparation time 13 mins Cooking Time forty-five mins
Servings twelve persons
Nutritional facts 267.4 calories Carb 40.1 gm Protein 5.5 gm Fat 9.1 gm Sodium 84.9 mg Potassium 140.89 mg Phosphorous 57.66 mg
Ingredients

- Unsalted, unprocessed, and half a cup of margarine
- Baking soda, 3/4 teaspoon
- One tablespoon of dissolved unsalted, unrefined margarine
- White flour, 5 cups
- Water, 2 1/4 cups
- Cream of tartar, two teaspoons

Instructions

- Set your oven's temperature to 350 º F.
- In a sizable mixing container, mix all of the dry Ingredients simultaneously.
- Put liquid and margarine or oil into the centre of the flour, filling the well. Stir it in slowly using a spoon or fork.
- As more liquid is included, a tender dough ball will eventually develop. You might need to include more liquid or flour as you whisk.
- To knead the bread and then pat it into a bread pot, create sure there is enough flour on the side of the container.
- In the container, knead the dough for around a min.
- In your preferred bread pot, flatten the dough.
- Create a cross on the bread and then slice it into pieces. The depth of the cut is around 14 inches.
- Bake for around 45 mins, or until the top and sides are golden brown.
- From the oven, remove. Spread margarine on the top to create it tenderer.
- Prior to wrapping with a fresh dish towel, let it cool.

58. Sweet Crustless Quiche.

Preparation time eighteen mins Cooking Time, one hr twenty mins
Servings six persons
Nutritional facts 219 calories Carb 25.7 gm Protein 5.5 gm Fat 11.1 gm Sodium 109.2 mg Potassium 199.46 mg Phosphorous 98.9 mg

Ingredients
- a half-cup of flour
- Three big eggs
- Brown sugar, 2 tablespoons
- Sliced or diced versions of three moderate apples
- Butter, 1/4 cup
- 1 cup of milk, 2%

Instructions
- Crack the eggs into a mixing dish and whisk in every component, dairy first, then flour, until most lumps are gone. Put the spices, salt, and pepper in if using.
- Cook the filling Ingredients in a griddle over moderate heat for 15-20 mins, or until well cooked and bubbling.
- A deep-dish pie plate or an 8-inch cake pot should be generously sprayed with cooking spray because the quiche will stick if it isn't. Cooked filling should be put halfway into a greased baking pot, then tenderly spread to distribute evenly. Bake at 350 º F for 40 to 45 mins, or until the top is golden brown and a knife inserted in the centre comes out clean.

59. Fruit & Cottage Cheese Omelet

Preparation time 3 mins Cooking Time two mins
Servings one person
Nutritional facts 216 calories Carb 13 gm Protein 19 gm Fat 10 gm Sodium 128 mg Potassium 258 mg Phosphorous 208 mg

Ingredients
- Low sodium cottage cheese, one-fourth cup
- drained half a cup of fruit salad from a can
- 1/9 cup of water
- two hens
- Sugar for icing (optional)

Instructions
- The eggs and water should be mixed in a small container.
- Coat an 8-inch (20-cm) nonstick griddle with cooking spray. Set the griddle's burner to moderate-high. In the pot, put the egg mixture. As the eggs set around the perimeter of the griddle, gently push the cooked sections towards the center using a spoon. Tilt and rotate the griddle to allow the raw egg to flow into open areas.
- When the eggs are nearly set on the surface but still appear moist, evenly spread cottage cheese across the center of the omelet. Put a quarter cup of fruit salad on top of the cottage cheese. Put the folded omelet on top of the fruit salad.
- The omelet should be taken out of the pot and put on a plate. If preferred, top with 1/4 cup of fruit and icing sugar..

60. Peach Raspberry Smoothie

Preparation time 3 mins Cooking Time zero mins
Servings 3 persons
Nutritional facts 129 calories Carb 23 gm Protein 6.3 gm Fat 3.2 gm Sodium 53 mg Potassium 261 mg Phosphorous 72 mg

Ingredients
- One tablespoon of honey, or sweeten with stevia or Splenda instead.
- frozen raspberries, one cup
- 1 moderate peach, pit taken out, and slices

- Unfortified almond milk, one cup
- a half-cup of tofu

Instructions

- Mix all of the components inside mixer till smooth.

61. Fresh Berry Fruit Salad with Yogurt Cream

Preparation time 7 mins Cooking Time zero mins
Servings eight persons
Nutritional facts 117 calories Carb 27 gm Protein 3.7 gm Fat 0.4 gm Sodium 40 mg Potassium 252 mg
Phosphorous 90 mg
Ingredients

- Blackberries, 1 cup
- a half-cup of honey
- Blueberries, 1 cup
- Greek yoghurt in two cups
- 1 cup of pitted and halved red cherries
- 1/4 cup honey
- Raspberry fruit, one cup
- Lemon juice, one tablespoon

Instructions

- In a mixing container, mix the berries and honey.
- In a another container, mix the components for the yoghurt cream.
- Every plate should have a dollop of yoghurt cream in the centre, followed by a berry fruit salad.

62. Spicy Pina Colada Smoothie

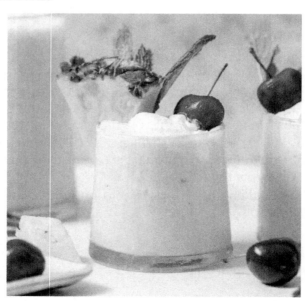

Preparation time 6 mins Cooking Time zero mins
Servings two persons
Nutritional facts 189 calorie Carb 32 gm Protein 13.4 gm Fat 5 gm Sodium 5 mg Potassium 349 mg
Phosphorous 121 mg
Ingredients

- Stevia or another sweetener, one teaspoon

- 12 cup of unsweetened pineapple juice
- One cup of tinned or fresh pineapple
- 1 cup (8 ounces) of firm tofu
- Red pepper flakes in one pinch

Instructions
- Simply create a puree of all the components inside a mixer.

63. Blueberry Smoothie

Preparation time 3 mins Cooking Time zero mins
Servings three persons
Nutritional facts 155.4 calories Carb 31.1 gm Protein 7.4 gm Fat 0.75 gm Sodium 104.1 mg Potassium 289.4 mg Phosphorous 27.5 mg
Ingredients
- Two teaspoons of Splenda or sugar
- Juice from one and a half cups of pineapple
- egg whites pasteurized in 1/4 cup
- water in a half-cup
- 2 cups of barely thawed frozen blueberries

Instructions
- Put all of the components inside a mixer.
- And puree.

64. Apple Mint French toast

Preparation time 3 mins Cooking Time eight mins
Servings two persons
Nutritional facts 352 calories Carb 60 gm Protein 12 gm Fat 8 gm Sodium 164 mg Potassium 40 mg Phosphorous 145 mg
Ingredients
- Mint, 1/8 teaspoon
- two eggs, mildly beaten
- Apple sauce, 1/4 cup
- Bread, four slices of white
- 1/2 cup milk

Instructions
- In a mixing container, mix milk, eggs, and mint.
- In a mixing basin, mix the rest of the components with the applesauce.
- Melt a little amount of margarine in a nonstick pot over a moderate-high temperature.
- Slices of bread are put in the pot after being dipped in the batter.
- Flip the bread over and continue cooking the second side until the lower part has browned.
- Include a drizzle of maple syrup finish.

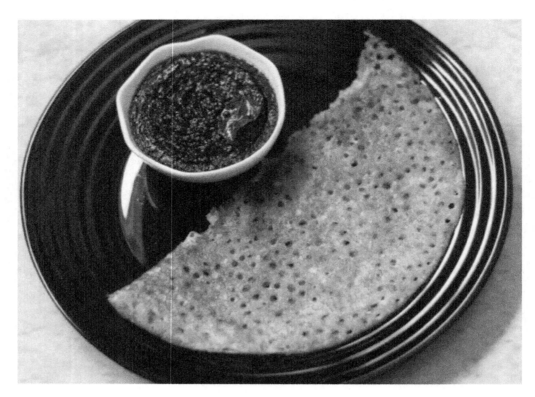

The lunch recipes are best for all people with kidney disease or impaired kidneys.

1. Renal-friendly Chicken Tikka

Preparation time 20 mins Cooking Time 70 mins
Servings four persons
Nutritional facts 176 calories Carb 12 gm Protein 5 gm Fat 5 gm Sodium 126 mg Potassium 171 mg
Phosphorous 99 mg
Ingredients

- 2 skinless, boneless chicken breasts
- Yoghurt low in fat (3 tbsp.)
- (1 tablespoon) curry paste
- (1 teaspoon) lemon juice

Instructions

- Curry paste and yoghurt should be mixed.
- In a container, layer the chicken with the yogurt-curry mixture, then top with the lemon. By letting it sit for an hr or even overnight, you can allow the flavours to merge.
- The chicken is heated, then grilled. It should take close to 20 mins for the meat to become juicy.
- Serve it with lettuce that has been sliced or in a tortilla wrap.
- Serve it as the main entrée with hot rice.

2. Apple Cranberry Walnut Salad

Preparation and Cooking Time one hr forty-five mins
Servings three persons
Nutritional facts 94 calories Carb 15.7 gm Protein 1 gm Fat 3.5 gm Sodium 61 mg Potassium 102 mg Phosphorous 26 mg
Ingredients

- 4 celery stalks, cut into quarter-inch sections
- Fat-Free Cranberry Balsamic Dressing, 8 ounces bottle
- One and a half cups of Ocean Spray (infused with pomegranate)
- Dried Cranberries, 1 package (6 ounces)
- 7 moderate-sized Gala Apples with the skin.
- 2 cups of seedless red grapes, every grape split in half.
- 1 13 cups of walnut halves, broken into little bits.

Instructions

- Red grape cluster should be washed and stem should be separated. Cut every grape into half with a paring knife. Put grapes inside a very big-sized mixing container and cut into slices.
- Half a walnut should fit into the measuring cup. You can either use a nut grinder or put the walnuts inside a plastic sandwich zip lock bag, seal it, and gently press the walnuts with the lower part of a cup measure to tear them into pea-sized bits. Include sliced nuts to the extra-big mixing container containing the red grape slices.
- To the mixture of grapes and walnuts, include one six-ounces bag of the dried cranberries infused with pomegranate.
- To the mixture of walnuts, grapes, and dried cranberries, include the washed, washed, and sliced celery into quarter-inch chunks.
- Seven Gala apples should be washed prior to being cut in 1/2 vertically & hollowed. Create five apples' wedges & then cut every wedge into bite-sized pieces. To the rest of the combination, include the sliced pieces of apple.
- Over the entire mixture, put the cranberry dressing from the eight-fluid ounce bottle. Create sure to mix the dressing and coat all of the components as you stir the Ingredients. Serve chilled.

3. Baked Salmon with Roasted Asparagus on Cracked Wheat Bun

Preparation time fifteen mins Cooking Time 30 mins
Servings three persons
Nutritional facts 394 calories Carb 23 gm Protein 35 gm Fat 18 gm Sodium 273 mg Potassium 976 mg Phosphorous 389 mg
Ingredients

- One tbsp. of olive oil
- 16 oz. of fresh salmon fillet
- One tbsp. of butter
- 12 oz. of fresh asparagus spears (woody stems discarded), washed
- One tbsp. of lemon juice
- 4 cracked whole-grain or wheat hamburger buns, toasted

Instructions

- Set the oven at 400 °F.
- Spray some olive oil on a cookie sheet and include the asparagus spears.
- Cook for 10 mins, or till tender and just beginning to flip brown.
- Take it out of your oven and then let it cool.

4. Roasted Asparagus and Wild Mushroom Stew

Preparation time 45 mins Cooking Time thirty mins
Servings four persons
Nutritional facts 103 calories Carb 12 gm Protein 3 gm Fat 6 gm Sodium 79 mg Potassium 437 mg
Phosphorous 70 mg

Ingredients

- one tbsp. of fresh sliced parsley
- ⅛ tsp. of onion powder
- 2 cups of vegetable stock, low sodium
- 1 carrot stick
- 2 oz. of pine nuts
- one tbsp. + one tsp. of dry Marsala wine
- 1 bay leaf
- ⅛ tsp. of garlic powder
- 1 small onion
- 1 cup of very hot water
- 1 fennel (anise) head
- ground black pepper as required
- 1 oz. of dried wild mushroom medley
- 4 sprigs of fresh thyme
- 2 tsps. of olive oil
- 1 lb. of asparagus
- 2 celery stalks
- 1 tsp. of dried sage
- pinch of cayenne pepper

Instructions

- Heat the oven to 400 F. It is advisable to wash and trim the rough lower parts off asparagus spears.
- Spread out the asparagus stalks in a single layer on a baking sheet. the spears with olive oil spray. Bake in the oven for 10 mins. Once the spears have cooled, cut them into 1-inch pieces.
- Reconstitute dried mushrooms in one cup of scalding hot water.
- A nonstick sauce pot is filled with celery, fennel, onions, carrots, and 1 teaspoon of olive oil, and it is cooked over moderate-high heat until the onions are translucent. You need to include the sage, garlic powder, thyme, cayenne pepper, marsala wine, sliced parsley, bay leaf, and onion powder and stir continuously for an additional min over flame. Include vegetable stock, the liquid from the dried mushrooms, and the diced wild mushrooms; simmer for 15 mins.
- Asparagus pieces, stew, and pine nuts should all be arranged in the dish starting at the lower part.

5. Baked Turkey Spring Rolls

Preparation time 45 mins Cooking Time forty-five mins
Servings six persons
Nutritional facts 197 calories Carb 10 gm Protein 23 gm Fat 7 gm Sodium 83 mg Potassium 323 mg Phosphorous 222 mg
Ingredients

- 2 teaspoons of ground black pepper
- 20 oz. of the 99% lean turkey breast (ground)
- 6 frozen spring roll pastry wrappers
- Non-stick cooking spray
- 2 ½ cups of coleslaw mix

- 2 tablespoons of minced cilantro
- 1 tablespoon of balsamic vinegar
- 2 tablespoons of vegetable oil
- 1 tablespoon of sesame oil

Instructions

- Set oven at 400° F.
- Spring roll wrappers should be removed from freezer and permitted to thaw at the room temp for around thirty mins prior to using.
- Raw turkey should be mixed with sesame oil, balsamic vinegar, & minced cilantro.
- A big-sized griddle should be coated with two tablespoons of vegetable oil. Then the griddle should be warm up on moderate-high flame. Now ground turkey should be included to heated griddle and stirred to crumble and then sauté till cooked.
- Then coleslaw mix should be included to the turkey on your griddle and cooking should be continued with intermittent stirring for five mins. Now two teaspoons of the ground black pepper should be sprinkled on the mixture and mixed well.
- It should be removed from flame & put away.
- Leaving space at both ends, near one corner of spring roll wrapper, distribute three tablespoons of the stuffing mixture diagonally. Over the filling, fold up the side closest to you, then create a tight roll by folding in both sides. To seal, dab some water on one of the wrapper's edges.
- Continually use the rest of the wrappers to repeat.
- Mildly mist a baking pot with nonstick cooking spray.
- A baking pot should be lined with spring rolls. Put it inside the oven & bake at 400°F for 30 mins.
- Serve as a dipping sauce with the sweet chili sauce.

6. Balsamic Marinated Mushrooms

Preparation time 15 mins Cooking Time, two hrs
Servings four persons
Nutritional facts 29 calories Carb 5 gm Protein 2 gm Fat 0.2 gm Sodium 7 mg Potassium 203 mg Phosphorous 51 mg
Ingredients

- One tablespoon of sliced chive + extra for the garnish
- Twelve button mushrooms, stems discarded
- ¼ cup of apple cider vinegar
- Quarter cup of balsamic vinegar
- Pinch of ground black pepper

Instructions

- The mushrooms should be put with the rest of the components inside a moderate-sized container and covered.
- Hands should be used for mixing everything simultaneously and then they should be put in the fridge for around two hrs.
- The mushrooms should be taken out of the container and separated them from the vinegar, and sprinkled with extra chives prior to serving.

7. Savory Kidney-Friendly Chicken and Dumplings

Preparation time 15 mins Cooking Time fifteen mins
Servings six persons
Nutritional facts 283 calories Carb 26.8 gm Protein 14.3 gm Fat 13 gm Sodium 186 mg   Potassium
478.6 mg Phosphorous 282.7 mg
Ingredients

- green beans, trimmed and diced into 1-inch pieces, amounting to 1/3 pound.
- Three Sriracha sauce drops
- Celery seed, 1/4 teaspoon
- 3 cups of chicken broth low in salt
- rosemary, half a teaspoon
- 1 1/2 cups of cooked chicken dice.
- divided into 5 tablespoons of cold, unsalted butter
- Thyme, half a teaspoon
- As required pepper Optional spices
- Fresh parsley, sliced, as required, plus more for the topping, 2 tbsp
- Bay leaf, one
- Baking powder, one tsp.
- 2 moderate-sized diced carrots
- 1 celery stalk, finely sliced divided
- 1/4 cups of all-purpose flour
- 1 teaspoon parsley
- 1/2 cup of rice milk or unsweetened almond milk
- 1 small yellow onion, minced

Instructions

- Three tablespoons of butter should be dissolved in a big pot on moderate-high heat. Cook for around 4 mins, or until the celery, onion, and carrots are transparent.
- Cook for one min while stirring constantly. As you include the broth, continue to stir as you bring to a boil. Lower the flame and cook for around 5 mins. After including the green beans, chicken, and spices, season with salt and pepper.
- The steps of making dumplings are as follows: In a mixing dish, mix 1/2 teaspoon coarse salt, 1 cup of flour, baking powder, and 2 tablespoons of parsley. Include almond milk and two teaspoons of butter that have been cut. Using a big spoon, you must heapingly drop spoonfuls of batter on top of the chicken mixture. Cook the dumplings for a further 12 mins, covered, or until thoroughly heated. Include extra parsley, sliced, to the serving dish.

8. Chicken and Gnocchi Dumplings

Preparation time fifteen mins Cooking Time forty-five mins
Servings ten persons
Nutritional facts 362 calories Carb 38 gm Protein 28 gm Fat 10 gm Sodium 121 mg Potassium 485
mg Phosphorous 295 mg
Ingredients

- A quarter cup of sliced fresh parsley
- 2 pounds of chicken breast
- ½ cup of finely diced fresh carrots
- One pound of gnocchi
- 1 teaspoon of black pepper
- A quarter cup of light olive or grapeseed oil
- 1 tablespoon of Better Than Bouillon Low Sodium Chicken Base
- 12 cups of fresh onions, diced finely
- 6 cups of chicken stock with less sodium
- a half cup of fresh celery, sliced finely One teaspoon of Italian seasoning

Instructions

- Put the stockpot on the stovetop, include the oil, and flip the flame around high.
- Cook the chicken in a hot griddle till golden brown on all sides.
- Continue to cook with the chicken till the carrots, celery, and onions are translucent. Cook for 20–30 mins on high flame with chicken stock.
- Diminish flame to low and mix in the black pepper, chicken bouillon, and Italian seasoning. Cook, stirring constantly, for 15 mins after including the gnocchi.
- Remove from the flame, garnish with parsley, and serve.

9. Rava Dosa: Low Sodium and Low Potassium Version

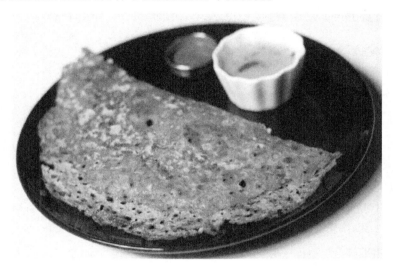

Preparation time ten mins Cooking Time thirty mins
Servings six persons
Nutritional facts 72 calories Carb 15 gm Protein 2 gm Fat 1 gm Sodium 131 mg Potassium 47 mg Phosphorous 65 mg
Ingredients

- 1/4 Cup of preferably sour Dahi or Yogurt
- 1 Green Chili
- A quarter Cup of Rava
- 1/4 Cup of Rice Flour
- A half tsp. of Cumin
- 1 Cup of Water
- One tsp. of Amchur

Instructions

- To create a coarse paste, crush half teaspoon of jeera and one green chili. The introduction of the green chili is completely optional.
- Insert in a big-sized container a quarter cup of rava (semolina), a quarter cup of rice flour, a quarter cup of yogurt or dahi (sour preferred), green chili-cumin paste, one teaspoon of Amchur (powder of dried mango), and 1/4 teaspoon of salt.
- Mix thoroughly.
- Insert 1/2 cup of water gradually and thoroughly mix.
- Allow 30 mins for the batter to rest. This is just to allow the rava to tenderen; otherwise, the dosa will be grainy.
- Because rava has soaked up the water, the batter will have thickened after 30 mins.
- Insert a little less than half cup water at a time, combining well after every introduction. The batter must be thin and easily available.
- Use quarter teaspoon oil to coat the surface of a 10″ nonstick tava (pot).

- Warm the pot till it is extremely hot. It really should sizzle and evaporate if you drop a water drop on it.
- The quarter cup batter, put into a cup, should cover the whole surface. It's not a great idea to try to spread out the batter.
- Flip the flame down to moderate.
- Cook the dosa till the edges begin to brown.
- Remove the dosa out from the tava's surface with a spoon. Loosen the edges as well as work your way towards the center.
- Flip the dosa over and cook for another two or three mins.
- To prepare the rest of the dosas, repeat the process.
- Serve the Rava Dosa with the Cranberry Chutney or on its own.

10. Leached Mashed Potatoes with Roasted Garlic

Preparation time 20 mins Cooking Time, 35 mins
Servings four persons
Nutritional facts 223 calories Carb 36 gm Protein 5 gm Fat 7 gm Sodium 42 mg Potassium 818 mg Phosphorous 135 mg
Ingredients

- One Tbsp. of olive oil
- 2 big potatoes peeled and diced
- parsley for garnish
- 1/4 cup of milk
- black pepper as required
- 1 Tbsp. of butter
- chives for garnish
- 1 head of garlic

Instructions

- Warm up your oven at 400 º F.
- Fill the pot halfway with cool water as well as bring to the boil.
- In the meantime, slice the top off the garlic head to expose the cloves and drizzle with olive oil. Put in the oven after wrapping in aluminum foil. Roast for thirty min, or till golden brown and tendered.
- When the potatoes have reached a boil, drain the water and replace it with enough amount of water to cover the potatoes. Bring to the boil once more, then cook till the potatoes are tender. Drain the water completely. Include the milk, butter, and garlic as required.
- Potatoes should be mashed. You can season using pepper as per taste. Serve with chives or parsley as a garnish.

11. Triple Berry

Preparation time three mins Cooking Time five mins
Servings one person
Nutritional facts 191 calories Carb 40.9 gm Protein 4 gm Fat 3.5 gm Sodium 143 mg Potassium 679 mg Phosphorous 76.6 mg
Ingredients

- A handful of baby spinach
- 1/4 cup of raspberries
- A half cup of almond milk
- 1/4 cup of blackberries
- A half cup of strawberries

Instructions

- Strawberries, blackberries, and a handful of baby spinach go into the mixer.
- Two cups of almond milk or coconut milk should be included to the mix.
- Blend till smooth and the desired smoothie texture has been achieved.
- Serve the smoothie in a glass with some extra fresh sliced strawberries as a garnish. It's time to drink.

12. Roasted Cauliflower, Carrots & Onions

Preparation time ten mins Cooking Time forty mins
Servings twelve persons
Nutritional facts 50 calories Carb 6 gm Protein 1 gm Fat 2 gm Sodium 30 mg Potassium 230 mg Phosphorous 23 mg
Ingredients

- One onion, sliced into big cubes
- Half head of cauliflower, sliced into small florets
- One tbsp. of olive oil
- 2 sliced carrots

Instructions

- Set your oven's temperature to 350 ⁰ F.
- Put the cauliflower, carrots, and onion in a single layer on a big baking sheet.
- Put oil over and stir to coat evenly.
- Set your oven to 400 ⁰ F, roast for 40 mins, and stir halfway through.
- Use seasonings like Herbs de Provence to enhance your food, such as herbs and spices.

13. Vegetarian Red Beans and Rice

Preparation time 1day Cooking Time two hrs thirty mins
Servings 12 persons
Nutritional facts 255 calories Carb 46 gm Protein 10 gm Fat 3.7 gm Sodium 188 mg Potassium 466 mg Phosphorous 170 mg
Ingredients

- 1 green bell pepper sliced fine
- 1 lb. of small dried red beans picked over & washed
- 1/2 tsp. of black pepper
- 1 bunch of sliced green onions
- 2 bay leaves
- 1 tbsp. of red wine vinegar
- 2 tsps. of smoked paprika
- 3 tbsps. of unsalted butter
- 2 celery stalks sliced fine
- 3/4 tsp. of salt
- 2 chipotles in adobo sauce sliced fine
- 1/8 tsp. of cayenne pepper
- 2 tsps. of dried thyme
- 1 onion sliced fine
- 4 cloves of garlic sliced
- 2 cups of white rice dry

Instructions

- The beans should soak for around 24 hrs. In a sizable mixing basin, mix the dried beans and four quarts (8 cups) of water. Give the soak around 12 hrs, but no more than 24. Wash the beans completely.
- Butter should be dissolved in a big soup pot or Dutch oven. After that, include celery, onion, bell pepper, and 1/2 teaspoon of salt. Cook the vegetables for around seven mins, or until they are tender.
- At this point, include the garlic, cayenne, chipotles, bay leaves, paprika, thyme, and black pepper. Cook until aromatic, which should take around 30 secs.
- 9 cups of water and the beans should be included to the pot. Heat the water until it boils. Cook for 45 mins, or until the liquid starts to cream up or thicken.
- Include the rest of the 1/4 teaspoon of salt and the vinegar. Cook the sauce for a further 30 mins, or until it is completely thick and creamy.
- Cook the rice as directed on the packet in the interim. Leave out the salt, butter, and oil.
- Serve 1/2 cup of cooked rice with 1/2 cup of beans. Serve garnished with a lot of green onions.

14. Stuffed Green Peppers/Kidney Friendly

Preparation time twenty-five mins Cooking Time one hr twenty mins
Servings twelve persons
Nutritional facts 259 calories Carb 20 gm Protein 16 gm Fat 12 gm Sodium 152 mg Potassium 313 mg Phosphorous 132 mg
Ingredients

- 4 tsps. of unsalted margarine, divided
- 1 tsp. of onion powder
- 1 1/2 tsps. of paprika
- 6 green peppers
- 1 tsp. of garlic powder
- 1 1/2 tsps. of poultry seasoning
- A half tsp. of pepper
- 3 cups of cooked rice
- 1 cup of water
- 2 tsps. of Mrs. dash onion herb seasoning
- 1/2 cup of sliced onion
- 1 cup of tender white bread crumbs
- 2 pounds of ground beef or turkey
- 6 tablespoons of mild thick and chunky style salsa

Instructions

- Remove the tops of the peppers and clean the insides. You can also clean out the insides of peppers by slicing them in half lengthwise.
- Then parboil for four mins.
- Cook ground beef till fully cooked inside big-sized frying pot. Drain all drippings from the meat into a coriander as well as keep it there till ready to use.
- The onion should be sautéed in 1 teaspoon of margarine until it is cooked and transparent.
- In a sizable mixing container, mix salsa, Mrs. Dash herb seasoning, onion powder, cooked rice, garlic powder, pepper, and meat. Stir everything simultaneously to blend.
- Bake green peppers in a shallow baking pot after stuffing them with a pork and rice combination. Put the peppers in the pot and halfway fill it with water.
- In a sizable mixing basin, mix the bread crumbs, dissolved margarine, and chicken spice.
- Over the stuffed peppers, sprinkle.

- Following that, roast the peppers in the oven at 350 º for 40 to 60 mins, or until fully cooked (time varies depending on whether you slice the peppers' tops off or cut them in half lengthwise).
- Remove the lid after the peppers are fully cooked and continue cooking for an additional 5 mins to brown the tops.

15. Kidney Bean and Cilantro Salad with Dijon Vinaigrette.

Preparation time fifteen mins Cooking Time fifteen mins
Servings four persons
Nutritional facts 154 calories Carb 18.3 gm Protein 5.5 gm Fat 7.4 gm Sodium 6 % Potassium 9 %
Phosphorous 8 %
Ingredients
- 1 tsp. of sumac
- 1 15-oz. can of kidney beans, drained & washed
- 1 bunch of fresh cilantro, sliced & stems removed (around 1 ¼ cups)
- 1 tsp. of Dijon mustard
- 1 sliced red onion
- 1 big lime or lemon, juice of
- Three tbsps. of extra virgin olive oil
- ½ tsp. of fresh garlic paste, or finely sliced garlic
- Salt & pepper, as required
- ½ sliced English cucumbers
- 1 sliced Moderate-sized heirloom tomato
Instructions
- Mix the sliced vegetables, kidney beans, and cilantro inside a moderate-sized mixing container.
- To create the vinaigrette, stir simultaneously the fresh garlic, sumac, oil, lime juice, mustard, and pepper inside a separate small-sized container.
- With a big-sized spoon, mix the vinaigrette into the salad thoroughly. If necessary, season using salt & pepper.
- Refrigerate for thirty mins to sixty mins prior to serving, covered.

16. Best Ever Guacamole (Fresh, Easy & Authentic)

Preparation time ten mins Cooking Time zero mins
Servings four persons
Nutritional facts 184.8 calories Carb 12.3 gm Protein 2.5 gm Fat 15.8 gm Sodium 305.5 mg Potassium
121 mg Phosphorous 78 mg
Ingredients
- 2 minced garlic cloves
- A half small onion, finely diced
- 3 ripe avocados
- 2 Roma tomatoes, diced
- One jalapeno pepper, seeds discarded and finely diced
- 1 juiced lime
- A half teaspoon of sea salt
- 3 tablespoons of finely sliced fresh cilantro
Instructions
- Cut the avocados, remove the pit, and scoop the contents into a mixing container.
- With a fork, mash the avocado till it is the desired amount of smooth or chunky.

- Mix the rest of the components inside a mixing container. Taste it and adjust the seasoning with a pinch of salt or lime juice if necessary.
- Guacamole is best served with tortilla chips.

17. Green Garden Salad

Preparation time ten mins Cooking Time zero mins
Servings three persons
Nutritional facts 87 calories Carb 4 gm Protein 1.5 gm Fat 8 gm Sodium 347 mg Potassium 204 mg Phosphorous 40 mg
Ingredients

- 2 pieces of celery stalks, sliced
- 4 cups of shredded red leaf or other lettuce
- 2 pieces of radishes, sliced
- 1 pc of big bell pepper, sliced or diced into rings
- Two pieces of cucumbers, sliced
- 1 piece of carrot, sliced

Instructions

- Mix the vegetables inside a big-sized container.
- Then whisk.
- You can serve with your favorite salad dressing.

18. Crunchy Lemon Herbed Chicken

Preparation time ten mins Cooking Time eighteen mins
Servings four persons
Nutritional facts 281 calories Carb 7 gm Protein 19 gm Fat 20 gm Sodium 63 mg Potassium 151 mg Phosphorous 123 mg
Ingredients

- 3 tablespoons of water (1 T for the egg wash, 2 T for the finishing of the sauce)
- 1 tablespoon of fresh sliced basil
- 4 tablespoons of unsalted butter (half chilled), divided
- Six pieces of green pepper, seeded with the tops removed
- 1 tablespoon of fresh sliced thyme
- 1/2 cup of Japanese bread crumbs (Panko)
- 6 pieces (2-oz.) of chicken tenders
- A half cup of cooked rice
- 1/4 cup of lemon juice, plus zest of one lemon
- 1 pc of egg yolk
- paprika
- 1 tablespoon of fresh sliced oregano

Instructions

- In a small saucepot, melt 2 tablespoons of butter over a low heat.
- Half of the herbs should be reserved for the lemon sauce; include one lemon's zest to the bread crumbs.
- Then mix egg yolk and one tablespoon water.
- The chicken tenders should be pounded between two pieces of plastic wrap until nearly ripped but not quite thin.
- Apply the egg wash mixture on the chicken first, and then the herbed-breadcrumb mixture.
- Flip up the heat to moderate-high and include the butter to the sauté pot containing the breaded chicken.
- The chicken should be cooked for two to three mins per side.

- Chicken should be taken out of the pot and put on a sheet tray to rest.
- Bring the water, additional herbs, and lemon juice to a gentle simmer in the same pot.
- Then extinguish the flame and vigorously whisk in the rest of the two tablespoons of cooled butter.
- Slice the chicken on the bias.
- Sliced chicken should be put on a platter, topped with sauce, and topped with the additional Ingredients.

19. Pasta with Pesto

Preparation time ten mins Cooking Time ten mins
Servings 8 persons
Nutritional facts 283 calories Carb 45 gm Protein 8 gm Fat 8 gm Sodium 45 mg Potassium 146 mg Phosphorous 115 mg
Ingredients
- 1 clove of garlic, minced
- A quarter cup of olive oil
- 1/4 cup of grated Parmesan cheese
- One lb. of pasta uncooked
- A quarter cup of sliced fresh parsley
- 2 tbsps. of dried basil

Instructions
- Inside a mixer or food processor, mix simultaneously all the components except pasta. Blend or process till the mixture is completely smooth.
- Cook pasta according to package directions in unsalted boiling water. Whisk the pasta with the sauce after it has been drained. Serve immediately.

20. Salisbury Steak

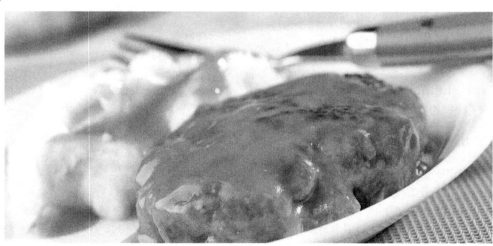

Preparation time ten mins Cooking Time twenty mins
Servings four persons
Nutritional facts 249 calories Carb 11 gm Protein 14.9 gm Fat 7 gm Sodium 128 mg Potassium 366 mg Phosphorous 218 mg
Ingredients
- 1 tablespoon of vegetable oil
- One teaspoon of black pepper
- 1 pound of sliced steak or lean ground beef, turkey or chicken
- A half cup of sliced green pepper
- 1 egg

- One small sliced onion
- 1 tablespoon of cornstarch
- A half cup of water

Instructions

- Mix the meat, egg, onion, green pepper, and black pepper inside a mixing container. Create patties out of the mixture.
- In a griddle, warm the oil, then include the patties as well as cook on both sides.
- Simmer for fifteen mins after including half of the water. Remove the patties from the pot.
- Include the rest of the water as well as cornstarch to the meat drippings. To thicken the gravy, continue to cook while stirring constantly.
- Serve the steak with gravy on top while it's still hot.

21. Korean-style Short Ribs

Preparation time twelve hrs thirty mins Cooking Time three hrs twenty-two mins
Servings six persons
Nutritional facts 286.7 calories Carb 2.4 gm Protein 21.9 gm Fat 20.4 gm Sodium 180.4 mg Potassium 309.04 mg Phosphorous 184.31 mg

Ingredients

- 1/2 bunch of finely sliced Green onions
- 2 Tbsps. of Soy sauce, low sodium
- 1 Tsp of Black pepper, ground
- ½ finely sliced Yellow onion
- 2 Tbsps. of White vinegar
- 1 1/2 lbs. of Beef Short Ribs
- 1/2 Cup of Water
- 2 Tbsps. of Rice wine vinegar
- 1 Tbsp. of Sriracha sauce
- 2 Tbsps. of granulated Sugar
- 4-6 Garlic cloves, finely sliced

Instructions

- Whisk simultaneously the soy sauce, Sriracha, water, sugar, vinegars, and pepper inside a big-sized mixing container. Mix the green onion, onion, and garlic inside a mixing container. To mix, stir everything simultaneously.
- Coat the short ribs in the marinade in a re-sealable plastic bag. To get a tight seal, remove as much air as possible from the bag. Allow for around twelve hrs of marinating time. (It would be preferable if you could give twenty-four hrs)
- Then use foil to cover a big-sized baking sheet. Remove the ribs from the marinade and discard the onions and garlic that remain on the ribs.
- Wrap the ribs in foil and bake for three hrs at 250°F. Remove the wrapper and serve.
- Serve with Jasmine or Basmati steamed rice.

22. Old Fashioned Canadian Stew

Preparation time thirty mins Cooking Time eight hrs
Servings eight persons
Nutritional facts 185 calories Carb 11 gm Protein 17 gm Fat 8.7 gm Sodium 153 mg Potassium 542 mg Phosphorous 184 mg

Ingredients

- 1 slice around 1.10 lbs. of the boneless beef blade, fat discarded
- 6 cloves of peeled garlic
- 4 cups of shredded cabbage

- 1 cup of sliced carrots
- 2 cups of turnip, cubed
- 1 tablespoon of mustard (whole-grain)
- 4 cups of low sodium beef or chicken broth
- 2 tablespoons of olive oil
- 1 cup of sliced onion

Instructions

- In a griddle with oil, sear the meat on the both sides. Put everything inside the slow cooker. Then put away.
- Brown the garlic and onion inside the same griddle.
- Include the mustard after deglazing with one cup of low salt beef or chicken broth. Put the rest of the Ingredients inside the slow cooker.
- Now cook for around eight hrs on low, or till the meat is fork-tender. Then season.

23. Asian Eggplant Dip with Seared Peppercorn Steak

Preparation time one hr five mins Cooking Time fifty-five mins
Servings twelve persons
Nutritional facts 131 calories Carb 7.3 gm Protein 17.4 gm Fat 3.2 gm Sodium 48 mg Potassium 386 mg Phosphorous 170 mg
Ingredients

- 2 tbsps. of sliced fresh cilantro
- 1 tbsp. of brown sugar
- 1 tsp. of sesame oil
- 2 tbsps. of brown sugar
- 1 tsp. of vegetable oil
- 4 finely sliced cloves of garlic
- 1 tsp. of chili paste
- 1 tbsp. of finely sliced fresh ginger root
- 4 sliced green onions
- 2 cloves of minced garlic
- 1 tsp. of olive oil
- 2 lbs. of sirloin steak
- 1 tbsp. of rice vinegar
- 1 big eggplant
- 1 tbsp. of cracked black peppercorns
- 1 tbsp. of water

Instructions

- Mix the Ingredients of marinade inside a small-sized container. Dry the steak, then brush it with oil and rub it with the mixture. Marinate for around an hr. Grill till desired level of doneness is reversed.
- Roast eggplant for 45 mins at 425°F in a warmed up oven.
- Peel the eggplant and finely slice it. Mix vinegar, sugar, and water inside a small-sized container. Garlic, green onions, ginger, and chili paste should be sautéed till fragrant in a big-sized griddle. Put in the vinegar mixture. When the sauce is bubbling, include the eggplant. To mix, stir everything simultaneously.
- Remove out of the flame and mix in the sesame oil. With grilled steak, serve cold or at room temperature.

24. Beef Thai Salad

Preparation time ten mins Cooking Time seventeen mins
Servings twelve persons
Nutritional facts 116 calories Carb 6 gm Protein 13 gm Fat 4.3 gm Sodium 77 mg Potassium 285 mg
Phosphorous 99 mg
Ingredients

- 1 tsp. of grated lime rind
- 1 tsp. of every Asian chili sauce and sesame oil
- 1/2 cup of halved grape tomatoes
- 1 lb. of Top Sirloin, Beef Strip Loin, or Flank Steak, finely sliced
- 8 cups of torn romaine lettuce
- ½ cup of EVERY julienned sweet yellow pepper, cucumber and red onion
- 1 tbsp. of cornstarch
- 1/4 cup of fresh lime juice
- 2 tbsps. of rice vinegar
- 1 tbsp. of EVERY liquid honey and sodium-diminished soy sauce, dash of Asian chili sauce
- 4 tsps. of canola oil
- 1 tbsp. of EVERY minced ginger root and fresh lime juice
- 2 cloves of garlic, minced

Instructions

- Mix the garlic, corn flour, sesame oil, ginger root, lime juice, and chili sauce in a moderate-sized mixing container. Include the beef, then leave it for 10 mins. Take out the marinade and throw it away.
- In the meantime, heat 1 tsp (5 ml) of canola oil in a big fry pot or wok over a moderate-high flame. Whisk the Ingredients in a clean container until they are heated and just starting to wilt. Stir-fry the meat in the same pot with the rest of the canola oil until it is done and browned. Mix by whisking in the wilting veggies.
- In a mixing container, mix all of the Ingredients for the chili-lime vinaigrette.
- In the pot, put the Chili-Lime Vinaigrette. Cook and stir until somewhat thickened and heated over moderate heat, scraping browned pieces from the pot's lower part. Include just enough hot vinaigrette to the romaine to create it wet. Over the romaine, spread the beef and vegetable combination. Drizzle the rest of the vinaigrette over every plate.

25. Oven Roast

Preparation time forty-five mins Cooking Time two hrs forty-five mins
Servings one person
Nutritional facts 122 calories Carb 12 gm Protein 23 gm Fat 3 gm Sodium 46 mg Potassium 241 mg
Phosphorous 154 mg
Ingredients

- Two pounds (1 kg) of oven Roast (Strip Loin, Prime Rib or Rib Roast)

Instructions

- Two-pound roast should be seasoned with pepper, rosemary, minced garlic, or thyme, if desired. Cover with a lid or cover and put in a dry, shallow roasting pot. Put a meat thermometer suitable for an oven in the roast's center, being careful not to touch the bone or fat.
- Sear the seasoned roast for 10 mins in a 450°F warmed up oven.
- Diminish at 275°F and roast to liked doneness; the meat is done when it reserves a temperature of 145°F to 170°F. Aim for 145°F if you prefer your roast at moderate-rare. If you prefer it well-done, aim for temperatures between 165- & 170-° F. It will take 1 hr. 45min (moderate rare) to 2 hr. 30min (well-done) to finish. When the temperature is 5°F below the finished temperature, take it out of the oven.
- Remove out of the oven, wrap loosely using foil, and set it aside for around 15 mins, or till the temperature has risen to around 5°F, prior to cutting into slices.

26. Classic Hamburgers

Preparation time eleven mins Cooking Time thirty-seven mins
Servings four persons
Nutritional facts 327.9 calories Carb 7.6 gm Protein 31.7 gm Fat 18.10 gm Sodium 162.8 mg Potassium 434 mg Phosphorous 225.9 mg
Ingredients

- 1 tsp. of no salt included steak spice (or ground pepper)
- 1 lb. of lean ground beef
- ¼ cup of dry bread crumbs
- 1 egg
- One tsp. of Dijon mustard
- 1 small onion, minced or 2 tbsps. of dried minced onion

Instructions

- Mix the bread crumbs, egg, spices, onion, and mustard inside a mixing container. Gently include and mix the beef. Form into patties (creates 4 regular sized burgers).
- Grill over moderate flame on a greased grill. Grill, flipping once, till the chicken's interior is no longer pink and the internal temperature reserves 160°F.

27. Pot Roast

Preparation time thirty-five mins Cooking Time four hrs forty-five mins
Servings ten persons
Nutritional facts 310 calories Carb 5 gm Protein 27 gm Fat 20 gm Sodium 62 mg Potassium 318 mg Phosphorous 219 mg
Ingredients

- 3 tablespoons of water, very cold
- 1 teaspoon of dried thyme
- 2 pounds of boneless beef chuck or rump roast
- 1 teaspoon of dried oregano
- 2 cups of water
- 1 cup of rutabagas (turnip)
- 3 table spoons of cornstarch
- 1/2 cup of sliced onion
- 3 garlic cloves, minced
- 2 tablespoons of vegetable oil
- Half cup of sliced carrots

Instructions

- In oil, brown the meat on all ends.
- Include the onions, cover, and cook for 15 mins on low flame.
- Include two cups water, rutabagas, garlic, and herb seasoning.
- Then simmer, covered for three and a half hrs to 4 hrs or till the meat is tender.
- Inside a small-sized container, mix simultaneously the cornstarch with cold water thirty mins prior to the pot roast is ready.
- To create slurry, include 1/2 cup of the hot liquid from the pot to the cornstarch mixture.
- Then reflip the mixture to the pot and stir it.
- Cook for another 30 mins after including the carrots.

28. Lemon Pepper Meatballs

Preparation time 16 mins & Cooking Time fifty mins

Servings six persons
Nutritional facts 358 calories Carb 3 gm Protein 30 gm Fat 23 gm Sodium 89 mg Potassium 301 mg
Phosphorous 151 mg
Ingredients

- 1/4 cup of finely sliced onion
- 1 teaspoon of garlic powder
- 3 tablespoons of lemon juice
- 1 tablespoon of vegetable oil
- 1/2 teaspoon of ground black pepper
- 1 teaspoon of cornstarch
- 1 tablespoon of sliced fresh parsley leaves
- 1 clove of garlic, minced
- 1 cup of water
- 2 pounds of lean ground beef
- 1 teaspoon of cold water
- 1/2 cup of fine, dry bread crumbs
- 1 big mildly beaten egg

Instructions

- Inside a moderate-sized mixing container, mix simultaneously the ground beef, garlic powder, bread crumbs, onion, egg, and pepper.
- Form 18 meatballs out of the mixture with moistened hands.
- Pot-fry the garlic and oil in a pot just big-sized enough to hold the meatballs in one layer for 5 mins over moderate low flame.
- Bring the water with lemon juice to the boil simultaneously.
- Cover and include the meatballs.
- Diminish to a low flame setting and cook for thirty min.
- With a slotted spoon, transfer the meatballs and keep them warm.
- Mix 1 tsp cold water as well as the cornstarch inside a small-sized container.
- Stir the cornstarch mixture into the broth mixture, then cook, stirring constantly, till the sauce has thickened.
- Remove the pot from the flame as well as stir in the parsley till everything is well mixed.
- Put the meatballs back in the pot and cook, stirring constantly, for one min over low flame.

29. Roast Beef with Yorkshire Pudding

Preparation time twenty mins Cooking Time one hr fifteen mins
Servings eight persons
Nutritional facts 251 calories Carb 9 gm Protein 27 gm Fat 11 gm Sodium 85 mg Potassium 405 mg
Phosphorous 262 mg
Ingredients

- Two eggs
- Beef tenderloin or other tender cut of beef (around 2 pounds)
- 1 cup of milk
- One cup of all-purpose flour
- Around quarter cup of vegetable oil for pot

Instructions

- Fresh herbs and black peppercorns are rubbed into the roast.

- For moderate doneness, roast beef at 350°F for around 20 mins per pound.
- After the roast has been removed from the oven, it will continue to cook mildly.
- Cover using aluminum foil and put away till ready to slice.
- To create the Yorkshire pudding, use a hand mixer to blend all of the components till smooth.
- Allow 30 mins for the mixture to chill.
- Warm up your oven at 425 ° F.
- Fill muffin tins' lower part with vegetable oil.
- Warm up the oven for around ten min, or till the oil is very hot in the oiled pot.
- Fill the muffin tins with the Yorkshire pudding mixture, around 3/4 full.
- Bake for 15 mins, or till golden and fluffy.

30. Fish Tacos

Preparation time eight mins Cooking Time sixteen mins
Servings eight persons
Nutritional facts 227.2 calories Carb 12.9 gm Protein 27.6 gm Fat 6.8 gm Sodium 99.3 mg Potassium 324.47 mg Phosphorous 235.01 mg
Ingredients
- Three tablespoons of flour, all purpose
- 8 Corn tortillas
- Lime wedges & lettuce for garnishing
- 2 lbs. of Cod fish
- 3 Tbsps. of Vegetable oil
- 1 Tbsp. of Chipotle powder
Instructions
- In a pot, warm the oil. Dredge the fish in flour and chipotle inside a container.
- Pot fry fish till it attains a temperature of 145 ° F.
- Warm tortillas in the oven wrapped in a tea towel.
- Serve the fish with lime juice squeezed over it.
- Serve with steamed vegetables or a Waldorf salad, green salad, or coleslaw.

31. Fish Cakes

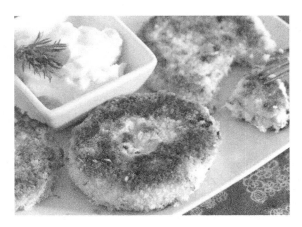

Preparation time thirteen mins Cooking Time seven mins
Servings eighteen persons
Nutritional facts 93 calories Carb 5.1 gm Protein 2.9 gm Fat 2.9 gm Sodium 82.7 mg Potassium 243.58 mg Phosphorous 139.35 mg
Ingredients

- Quarter tsp. of pepper
- Two lbs. of cod
- Three cups of bread crumbs
- 2 sliced small onions
- 1/4 cup of butter for cooking

Instructions

- Cut the fish into chunks and mix with the breadcrumbs, onions, and pepper inside a mixing container.
- Use a food processor to process the mixture.
- Form the ground mixture into patties; with 2 lbs. of fish, you should get around 18 fish cakes if the patties are 3 inches in diameter and 12 inches thick.
- Five mins on every side, fry the patties in butter.

32. Tuna Macaroni Salad

Preparation time seven mins Cooking Time eight mins
Servings eight persons
Nutritional facts 136 calories Carb 18 gm Protein 8 gm Fat 3.6 gm Sodium 75 mg Potassium 124 mg Phosphorous 90 mg
Ingredients

- Two diced celery stalks
- 1 1/2 cups of uncooked macaroni
- One Tsp. of lemon pepper seasoning
- 1/4 cup of mayonnaise
- One 170g can of tuna (white flaked or solid) packed in water

Instructions

- Cook the pasta and put it in the fridge to chill.
- Drain the tuna and wash it in a colander.
- When the macaroni is cool enough to handle, include the tuna and celery.
- Mix in the mayonnaise and lemon pepper.
- Chill prior to serving.

33. Jamaican Steamed Fish

Preparation time six mins Cooking Time fourteen mins
Servings four persons
Nutritional facts 276 calories Carb 6 gm Protein 21 gm Fat 31 gm Sodium 106 mg Potassium 432 mg Phosphorous 188 mg
Ingredients

- 3/4 cup of red and green peppers, sliced
- 4 fillets of tilapia (100 g per fillet)
- Juice of 1/2 Lime (1 tbsp. of lime juice)
- 1/4 tsp. of black pepper
- 1 tsp. of hot pepper sauce
- 1/2 cup of olive oil
- 1 cup of hot water
- 1/2 cup of onion, sliced
- 1 tbsp. of Ketchup
- 1 big sprig thyme

Instructions

- On moderate flame, sauté onion and bell peppers in oil in a frying pot.
- Stir in 1/2 cup hot water, ketchup, black pepper, thyme, hot pepper sauce, and lime juice.

- Put fish in pot with 1/2 cup hot water, then put vegetables and sauce.
- Cook for five min with the lid on the pot. Cook for another 5 mins, covered, or till fish is done.

34. Shrimp and Apple Stir Fry

Preparation time sixty mins Cooking Time twenty-seven mins
Servings four persons
Nutritional facts 152 calories Carb 8 gm Protein 8 gm Fat 12 gm Sodium 151 mg Potassium 219 mg
Phosphorous 130 mg
Ingredients

- 2 Celery stalks, diced
- 1/2 lb. of Headless shrimp with shells
- 2 tbsps. of Vegetable oil
- Dash of White pepper
- 1 tsp. of Cornstarch
- 1 tsp. of Sugar
- 1/2 tsp. of Low sodium soy sauce
- 1 tsp. of Cornstarch
- 1/2 Sweet red pepper, diced
- 3/4 Apple, diced
- 2 tbsps. of Cold water
- 1/2 tsp. of Low sodium soy sauce

Instructions

- Remove the shrimp's shells and devein them. For half an hr, marinate the shrimp in the marinade Ingredients.
- Inside a small-sized mixing container, mix the sauce Ingredients. Put away after thoroughly mixing.
- In a nonstick wok, warm around one tablespoon of oil. Remove the shrimp from the wok after they have flipped pink in color.
- In a nonstick wok, warm around one tbsp. of oil. Stir fry the celery for a few secs prior to including the diced apple and red pepper and cooking till almost done. Stir constantly till the sauce thickens after including the shrimp and the sauce mixture.

35. Tuna Spread

Preparation time four mins Cooking Time zero mins
Servings four persons
Nutritional facts 101 calories Carb 1.3 gm Protein 12.4 gm Fat 4.9 gm Sodium 37 mg Potassium 91 mg
Phosphorous 133 mg
Ingredients

- Half tsp. of Dijon mustard
- One can (170g) of no salt included tuna, drained
- One tsp. of lemon juice
- 2 Tbsps. of light mayonnaise
- Use pepper as required

Instructions

- Mix simultaneously all of the components into a container with a fork.
- It should be seasoned with pepper.
- Serve on crackers or toast.

36. BBQ lemon and dill salmon

Preparation time seven mins Cooking Time five-six mins
Servings four persons
Nutritional facts 282 calories Carb 2 gm Protein 22 gm Fat 20 gm Sodium 140 mg Potassium 300 mg Phosphorous 218 mg
Ingredients

- 1 Tbsp. of whole grain Dijon mustard
- 1/4 Cup of sliced fresh dill
- 1/4 tsp. of black pepper
- 4, 3 oz. of salmon filets, deboned
- 1 sliced lemon
- 4 Tbsps. of olive oil

Instructions

- Warm up the BBQ to moderate-high.
- Put every filet of salmon, fresh or frozen, on a piece of aluminum foil.
- Drizzle with one tbsp. extra virgin olive oil.
- Then include a quarter teaspoon of Dijon mustard, 1/4 cup of fresh dill, salt & pepper as required, and a few lemon slices.
- Wrap in aluminum foil, making sure the edges are well sealed.
- Over direct flame, include the salmon. It only takes around 5-6 mins for this, but only 4-5 mins for moderate.

37. Chili Aioli Shrimp Dip

Preparation time five mins Cooking Time zero mins
Servings nineteen persons
Nutritional facts 95 calories Carb 0.16 gm Protein 0.02 gm Fat 10.4 gm Sodium 74.8 mg Potassium 4.30 mg Phosphorous 0.57 mg
Ingredients

- One tsp. of lemon juice
- Half clove of minced garlic
- One tsp. of Thai chili sauce
- one to two Tbsps. of sliced parsley
- One cup of Hellman's mayo

Instructions

- Mix all of the components.
- You can dip shrimp cocktail in it.
- On a tomato sandwich, it can also be spread.

38. Asian Noodle Stir Fry

Preparation time five mins Cooking Time four mins
Servings four persons
Nutritional facts 331 calories Carb 38 gm Protein 14 gm Fat 13 gm Sodium 165 mg Potassium 335 mg Phosphorous 230 mg
Ingredients

- 2 tbsps. of oil for stir frying
- 200g of chow mein noodles (par-cooked using the Instructions on package)
- 6 finely sliced shiitake mushrooms
- 2 finely sliced scallions
- 1 leek shredded

- 2 tbsps. of pickled ginger
- Sesame oil
- 2 eggs beaten
- 3 tbsps. of mirin (rice cooking wine)
- 1 1/3 cups of bean sprouts
- Chili oil
- 12 raw tiger shrimp shelled & deveined
- 2 tbsps. of fresh cilantro leaves

Instructions

- Cook the noodles as per the package Instructions, then strain and put inside a container.
- Whisk the noodles with the leek, shrimp, mushrooms, bean sprouts, and eggs, and whisk well to mix.
- Warm a big-sized griddle or a wok over high flame with a little oil till very hot.
- Stir in the noodle mixture till golden brown and the shrimp are pink and cooked through.
- Whisk in the mirin and cilantro till well mixed.
- Distribute the noodles among four containers, drizzle with the chili and sesame oils, and top with scallions and ginger.

39. Salmon Rice Salad

Preparation time one hr twenty mins Cooking Time twenty mins
Servings four persons
Nutritional facts 236 calories Carb 22 gm Protein 8 gm Fat 13 gm Sodium 145 mg Potassium 183 mg
Phosphorous 130.5 mg
Ingredients

- ¼ cup of French dressing
- 1 tbsp. of finely sliced onion
- ½ cup of sliced celery
- ½ cup of salmon, low sodium, drained
- ½ cup of cucumber, sliced
- 1 tsp. of horseradish
- ½ tsp. of celery seed
- 1 sliced & cooked egg
- ½ cup of rice, uncooked
- ¼ tsp. of pepper

Instructions

- Put rice in a saucepot with two cups (500 ml) water to cook.
- Bring to the boil, covered. Diminish to a low flame and cook for around 15 to 20 mins, or till rice is tender.
- Remove from pot as well as put away for 15 mins, covered.
- Whisk the hot cooked rice with the French dressing.
- Permit to completely cool at the room temperature prior to including the rest of the Ingredients.
- Mildly mix the components.
- Prior to serving, chill for around one hr.

40. Shrimp, Sugar Snap Pea Salad and Wasabi-Lime Vinaigrette

Preparation time six mins Cooking Time three mins
Servings six persons
Nutritional facts 334 calories Carb 17 gm Protein 19 gm Fat 22 gm Sodium 119 mg Potassium 489 mg
Phosphorous 212 mg
Ingredients

- 2 cups of snap peas, trimmed
- 1 cup of bean sprouts
- 1/2 tsp. of ginger, minced
- 1 tsp. of sugar
- 1/2 cup of vegetable oil
- 1 tbsp. of lime juice
- 1/2 tsp. of garlic, minced
- 3 tsps. of wasabi powder
- 1 lb. of big shrimp, peeled
- 1/4 cup of rice wine vinegar
- 1 cup of water chestnuts, drained

Instructions

- A big-sized pot of water should be brought to the boil.
- Cook till the shrimp flip pink, then include the snap peas.
- To avoid further cooking, immediately transfer the shrimp as well as snap peas to iced water and strain.
- Mix the vinaigrette's components with a whisk.
- Serve with vinaigrette that includes shrimp, water chestnuts, snap peas, and bean sprouts.

41. Curried Shrimp Salad Rolls

Preparation time 4 mins Cooking Time 6 mins
Servings 1 person
Nutritional facts 131 calories Carb 24 gm Protein 8 gm Fat 1.20 gm Sodium 62 mg Potassium 399 mg
Phosphorous 114 mg
Ingredients

- basil, cilantro (as required)
- Four shrimps
- Two peach slices
- 1 tsp. of curry paste
- lettuce
- Rice Paper

Instructions

- Put away to cool after sautéing the shrimp in curry paste.
- Inside a container of warm water, soak rice paper.
- To absorb some of the moisture, put rice paper on a towel.
- Put shrimp, peach slices, Thai basil, cilantro, as well as lettuce on the rice paper.
- Roll tightly and serve with garlic-ginger dipping sauces or mint yogurt.

42. Eggplant and Tofu Stir-Fry

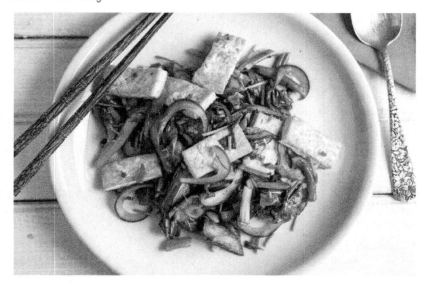

Preparation time seven mins Cooking Time fifteen mins
Servings four persons
Nutritional facts 374 calories Carb 36 gm Protein 16 gm Fat 20 gm Sodium 137 mg Potassium 250 mg Phosphorous 160 mg
Ingredients

- 4 tbsps. of canola oil
- 1 cup of long grain white rice
- 3 tbsps. of rice vinegar
- 1/4 cup of fresh basil leaves, torn
- 1 small eggplant
- 4 scallions sliced
- 1 package, 454g, of Tofu, cut into one-inch squares, moderate firm, and prepared with calcium sulfate
- 2 tbsps. of hoisin sauce
- 1 tsp. of cornstarch
- 1 red serrano or jalapeno pepper
- 2 sliced cloves of garlic

Instructions

- Cook rice as directed on the package.
- In a nonstick griddle, warm 1 tablespoon of oil. Whisk in the tofu and cook, flipping occasionally, for around 10 mins, or till golden brown. Put on a plate.
- Put in the rest of the oil. Cook till the vegetables are tender. Whisk in the sauce, then the tofu, and so on. Continue to whisk till the sauce has thickened. Serve with rice and basil on top.

43. Tilapia Tostadas with Corn-Zucchini Sauté and Basmati-Lime Pilaf

Preparation time nine mins Cooking Time twenty-five mins
Servings twelve persons
Nutritional facts 319 calories Carb 49 gm Protein 18 gm Fat 6 gm Sodium 50 mg Potassium 432 mg Phosphorous 199 mg
Ingredients

- One tbsp. of vegetable oil
- 12 six-inch white flour tortillas
- 1/2 cup of sliced cilantro

- 5 cups of water
- 3 cups of basmati rice
- 1 sliced green onion
- 2 tsps. of lime juice
- 1 garlic clove
- 1 tsp. of lime zest
- 2 cups of frozen corn
- 1 moderate sweet red pepper, diced
- One tsp. of red chili flakes
- 1 tbsp. of vegetable oil
- 2 diced moderate zucchini
- 1 tsp. of chili powder
- 4 (3-4 oz.) of tilapia fillets
- Three tbsps. of cilantro
- 1 tbsp. of vegetable oil

Instructions

- The Basmati-Lime Pilaf should be prepared first.
- Bring a pot of water to boil prior to including the rice.
- Cook, covered, for around 15 mins, or till the water has been absorbed.
- Mix the lime zest, lime juice, and cilantro inside a mixing container.
- Cover and put away to allow the flavors to mix.
- Warm up your oven at 350 º F.
- Mix the chili powder and the vegetable oil inside a container.
- Brush the flour tortillas with the chili oil. Bake them till crisp.
- Then in 1 tablespoon vegetable oil you need to sauté the onion and garlic.
- Cook till the tilapia is firm, stirring occasionally.
- Whisk the fish with cilantro that has been freshly sliced.
- Then put away.
- In a pot, warm the oil.
- Cook on high flame till the zucchini is tender, then include the vegetables.
- Then put away.
- On a plate, put a crisp tortilla.
- Arrange the rice, vegetable sauté, and fish in layers.
- Warm the dish prior to serving.

44. Crab Cakes

Preparation time six mins Cooking Time two mins
Servings eight persons
Nutritional facts 75 calories Carb 4 gm Protein 5 gm Fat 5 gm Sodium 88 mg Potassium 116 mg
Phosphorous 60 mg
Ingredients

- sliced fresh parsley
- 1/4 cup of diced red pepper
- 1 tsp. of lemon juice
- 120g of crab meat
- black pepper as required
- 1 sliced green onion
- 1 clove of garlic
- 1 egg

- vegetable oil
- 1/4 cup of bread crumbs

Instructions

- Mix all of the components inside a mixing container.
- The mixture should be divided into eight equal parts.
- Hand-form the crab cakes, ensuring that any excess liquid is squeezed out.
- Warm a frying pot over moderate-high flame and coat the lower part with enough vegetable oil.
- Cook the crab cakes in a griddle for around two mins on every side, or till golden brown.
- Serve right away.

45. Kidney-Friendly Chicken and Ginger Congee

Preparation time twelve mins Cooking Time fifty-eight mins
Servings four persons
Nutritional facts 339 calories Carb 41 gm Protein 21 gm Fat 6 gm Sodium 170 mg Potassium 332 mg
Phosphorous 222 mg

Ingredients

- 1 tbsp. of low-sodium oyster sauce
- ¾ cup of white rice
- 1 tsp. of low-sodium chicken powder
- 2 pieces of green onion
- 8 cups of water
- 2 tsps. of cornstarch
- 300 g of skinless chicken breast (or use any amount)
- 2 tbsps. of vegetable oil
- 1-inch of chunk peeled, fresh ginger
- 2 tbsps. of water

Instructions

- Inside a container, wash the rice by massaging and mixing it with your hands. Then remove the water and carry out the procedure three more times till the water is clear.
- Inside a big-sized pot, bring water to boil over high flame.
- Ginger should be finely sliced and then cut into strips. Green onion should then be sliced into small pieces.
- Cut the chicken into thin slices around 12 cm thick with a different cutting board and put it inside a container to marinate.
- Mix the chicken inside a container with the oyster sauce, chicken powder, cornstarch, and water for around 30 secs, or till there is no liquid left.
- Include the vegetable oil to the container and stir for another 30 secs with chopsticks. Set it aside for around 10-15 min to marinate.
- Once the water has raised to a boil, include the rice and gently stir it around the pot. Cover the pot using a lid & wait for it to boil again (around 2 mins.)
- After the pot comes back to the boil, partially cover it and diminish the flame to moderate to cook for 30 mins. Rice will adhere to the lower part of your pot if it is stirred.
- After 30 mins, rapidly and continuously whisk the rice for around 3-5 mins.
- Increase the flame to high & include the chicken in a slow, steady stream for 30-60 secs, stirring constantly. Wait for the pot to boil while stirring the chicken for another 1-two min.
- When the water begins to boil, include the ginger strips as well as season using salt. For around 20-30 secs, stir.

- Season using white pepper and stir till everything is well mixed. Serve with green onions as a garnish.

46. Za'atar Chicken with Garlic Yogurt Sauce

Preparation time twenty-three mins Cooking Time fifty-seven mins
Servings four persons
Nutritional facts 413 calories Carb 9.3 gm Protein 26.7 gm Fat 29.7 gm Sodium 118 mg Potassium 323.33 mg Phosphorous 196.73 mg
Ingredients

- 2 heads of Garlic, halved crosswise (5 cloves every)
- 4 Chicken thighs
- Black pepper, freshly ground – as required
- 1 tsp. of Lemon zest
- 1/cup of Extra Virgin Olive Oil
- 1 quartered Lemon, seeds removed
- 1/2 cup of Greek Yogurt, plain
- 1 tsp. of Lime zest
- 3 Tbsps. of Za'atar Spice Blend
- 1 tsp. of Coriander, ground
- 2 Spanish Onions, sliced in 1" wedges

Instructions

- Warm up your oven at 325°F. In a baking dish/roasting pot, arrange the chicken thighs, onions, garlic halves, and lemon quarters.
- Season using salt & pepper after putting in the oil. Coat all of the Ingredients in flour.
- Warm up your oven at 350°F and roast for 50 mins. The internal temperature must be around 175 º F.
- Meanwhile, inside a small-sized container, grate one garlic clove, include pepper, yogurt, and a splash of water to loosen the sauce.
- Remove the pot out of the oven & put away all but the chicken thighs.
- To crisp the skin, increase the temperature of your oven to 400 º F.
- Mix the pot drippings, lime zest, Za'atar seasoning, lemon zest, and pepper inside a mixing container.
- Chicken thighs should be rubbed with the mixture.
- Serve with sliced parsley or Lemon and Garlic Yogurt Sauce.

47. Lime Grilled Turkey

Preparation time two hrs Cooking Time six mins
Servings four persons
Nutritional facts 245 calories Carb 11.5 gm Protein 17.1 gm Fat 15 gm Sodium 35 mg Potassium 200 mg Phosphorous 131mg
Ingredients

- One tsp. of rosemary, dried
- A half cup of lime juice
- 2 tbsps. of honey, liquid
- ⅔ lb. of turkey breast, skinless & boneless
- One tsp. of thyme leaves, dried
- A quarter cup of vegetable oil

Instructions

- Mix the Ingredients to create the marinade.

- Two tbsps. (30 ml) marinade should be put away for basting.
- To create thinner pieces, cut the turkey breast in half lengthwise (like a hamburger bun is cut in half).
- Refrigerate the turkey for 1–2 hrs after including it to the marinade.
- Warm up the oven broiler to high (500°F).
- The turkey should be grilled or broiled for four mins per side till turkey is cooked through.
- To baste the turkey while it's cooking, use the marinade.
- Discard any leftover marinade.

48. One Pot Mediterranean Chicken & Pasta

Preparation time twenty-three mins Cooking Time twenty-six mins
Servings eight persons
Nutritional facts 245 calories Carb 26 gm Protein 21 gm Fat 4.4 gm Sodium 84 mg Potassium 436 mg Phosphorous 222 mg
Ingredients

- 1/2 tsp. of ground black pepper
- 2 moderate zucchini, raw, sliced
- 1/4 tsp. of rosemary, dried
- 2 moderate-sized chicken breasts, boneless & skinless, cut into bite-sized cubes
- 2 tsps. Of cornstarch
- 1 tsp. of basil, dried
- 2 tomatoes, diced
- 3 tbsps. of parmesan cheese, shredded
- 1 tbsp. of olive oil
- 2 cups of pasta, dry
- 1/2 tsp. of oregano, leaf, dried
- 2 1/2 cups of chicken broth, low sodium
- 3 garlic cloves, minced
- 1/2 cup of red or white wine
- 2 tbsps. of fresh parsley, sliced
- 1 moderate sweet red pepper, diced

Instructions

- Cut zucchini into half-moons by slicing it lengthwise. Tomatoes as well as red pepper should be diced into bigger pieces. Garlic should be minced. Set everything aside.
- Chicken breasts should be cut into bite-sized pieces (approximately 1 inch – 2.5 cm every).
- Warm the olive oil inside a big-sized pot over moderate-high flame for a min or two. Include the chicken and cook for around 10 mins, or till mildly browned. Stir once in a while.
- In the same pot, mix the zucchini, red peppers, tomatoes, and garlic. Include basil, rosemary, oregano, and black pepper as required. Stir and cook for 5-7 mins on moderate high flame, or till vegetables are crisp and tender. Remove the pot from the flame but leave it in the pot.
- In a separate pot, bring white wine and chicken broth to the boil over moderate high flame. To ensure even cooking, include the pasta and push it down with a spoon till it is completely submerged in the broth. Diminish flame to moderate and cook pasta as per the package Instructions, till al dente, as it will be heated further in the next step. To keep the pasta from sticking, stir it frequently while it's cooking.
- Remove one cup (250 ml) of the broth from the pasta pot and put away inside a moderate-sized container. Whisk in the cornstarch till no lumps remain.
- Whisk the chicken and vegetables with the rest of the liquid as well as cornstarch mixture. Stir and cook for a few mins over moderate flame or till sauce is thick.

- Sprinkle with shredded parmesan cheese prior to serving.

49. Persian Chicken

Preparation time sixty mins Cooking Time twenty mins
Servings ten persons
Nutritional facts 361 calories Carb 3 gm Protein 22 gm Fat 29 gm Sodium 86 mg Potassium 253 mg Phosphorous 159 mg
Ingredients

- Two tsps. of sweet paprika
- 1 big sliced onion
- A half cup of fresh lemon juice
- 2 tsps. of minced garlic
- One cup of olive oil
- 2 tbsps. of dried oregano
- Ten boneless & skinless chicken thighs

Instructions

- Puree the onion, paprika, oregano, lemon juice, and garlic inside the container of a mixer or food processor. Slowly put in the oil during the process.
- Drizzle the chicken with the marinade in a big, re-sealable plastic bag. Seal the bag tightly after pressing out the air. Refrigerate for 1 hr after flipping the bag to distribute the marinade.
- Remove the chicken from the marinade and whisk out any leftovers. Grill the chicken for around 10 mins over direct moderate flame, flipping once. Ascertain that there is no trace of pink inside and that the internal temperature is 165 º F. Serve alongside rice as well as a green salad.

50. Chicken in Mushroom Sauce

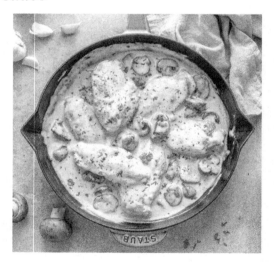

Preparation time thirteen mins Cooking Time eleven mins
Servings eight persons
Nutritional facts 161 calories Carb 5 gm Protein 25 gm Fat 4 gm Sodium 99 mg Potassium 289 mg Phosphorous 205 mg
Ingredients

- 2 tbsps. of light sour cream
- 1/4 cup of all-purpose flour
- 3 sliced green onions
- 1 1/2 cups of mushrooms, quartered
- Fresh ground pepper & sliced fresh parsley as required
- 1 cup of chicken broth

- 1 tbsp. of non-hydrogenated margarine
- 1 tbsp. of Dijon mustard
- 4 chicken breasts
- 1/4 tsp. of dried thyme

Instructions

- Two tablespoons sour cream, mustard, flour, and 2 tablespoons of chicken broth should be mixed first. Dredge the chicken in flour after seasoning it using thyme and pepper. In a big-sized nonstick griddle, melt margarine over moderate-low flame. You need to cook for around 5 mins per side, or till the chicken's interior is no longer pink. Remove the chicken from the pot and keep it warm.
- Fill the griddle with the mushrooms and cook for 3 mins, stirring occasionally. Increase the flame to high & cook for 3 mins with the rest of the chicken broth. Inside a separate container, whisk simultaneously the sour cream and green onions. Stir till the sauce has thickened (around 3 mins). Serve with pepper and parsley.

51. Chicken Stew with Mushrooms and Kale

Preparation time seven mins Cooking Time nine mins
Servings four persons
Nutritional facts 199 calories Carb 12 gm Protein 25 gm Fat 6 gm Sodium 94 mg Potassium 500 mg Phosphorous 254 mg
Ingredients

- 1/2 tablespoon of poultry seasoning
- 1/4 cup of diced onion
- 1/2 teaspoon of ground black pepper
- 1 tablespoon of cornstarch
- 1/2 teaspoon of paprika
- 1 cup of kale, washed, stemmed, & sliced
- 2 cups of homemade or no-salt included chicken stock
- 1 tablespoon of olive oil
- 1 clove of garlic, minced
- 1/2 cup of red pepper, sliced
- 1/2 cup of shitake mushrooms, washed, stemmed, & sliced
- 1/4 teaspoon of garlic powder
- 1/2 cup of milk
- 2 cups of cooked chicken (or turkey), sliced
- 1/2 cup of button mushrooms, washed, stemmed & sliced

Instructions

- In a big-sized griddle, sauté the onions and garlic till they tendered as well as the onions become translucent. Continue to sauté the rest of the vegetables till they tendered as well as the mushrooms begin to brown.
- Bring the vegetable mixture to a simmer with the chicken stock, cooked chicken, and dry spices.
- Mix the milk and cornstarch in a separate container and whisk till smooth. Stir into the simmering stew till it thickens.
- The stew is ready to eat once it has thickened. Serve with rice or noodles of your choice.

52. Chicken Dijon Marinade

Preparation time fifty mins Cooking Time twenty mins
Servings four persons
Nutritional facts 282.3 calories Carb 1 gm Protein 30 gm Fat 17 gm Sodium 134 mg Potassium 256 mg Phosphorous 209 mg

Ingredients

- Half a teaspoon of ground pepper
- Two Tbsps. of canola oil
- One pound of chicken (breasts or thighs)
- 1 Tbsp. of Dijon mustard

Instructions

- Mix all of the Ingredients simultaneously.
- Marinate the chicken.
- It should be grilled on med-high flame for approximately twenty mins (flipping once) or till it is no pinker.

53. Turkey Sliders with Peach Tarragon Aioli

Preparation time twelve mins Cooking Time eight mins
Servings three persons
Nutritional facts 257 calories Carb 4 gm Protein 16 gm Fat 11 gm Sodium 257 mg Potassium 330 mg Phosphorous 240 mg
Ingredients

- 1/2 tablespoon of Dijon mustard
- 450 g of ground turkey
- 2 tablespoons of peaches, pureed
- 1 teaspoon of poultry seasoning
- 1/4 cup of red onion, diced
- 6 slider buns
- 1/2 cup of arugula
- 1 teaspoon of garlic powder
- 1/3 cup of sliced parsley
- 1 teaspoon of sliced tarragon
- 2 tablespoons of mayonnaise

Instructions

- Warm up the grill pot or the BBQ to moderate/high flame. Mix the turkey, poultry seasoning, parsley, garlic powder, Dijon mustard, and red onion inside a mixing container. Create 6 patties out of the mixture.
- Cook the turkey sliders for 5-6 mins per side, or when the internal temperature reaches 165 ° F.
- Create peach tarragon aioli.
- Spread aioli on the top and lower part of the slider buns to create the turkey sliders. Top the lower part bun with a turkey patty. Garnish with arugula and put bun on the top.

54. Chicken Makhani

Preparation time nine mins Cooking Time forty-two mins
Servings four persons
Nutritional facts 214 calories Carb 22 gm Protein 9 gm Fat 11 gm Sodium 51 mg Potassium 419 mg Phosphorous 130 mg
Ingredients

- 2 tbsps. of oil
- 1 lb. of boneless, & skinless chicken thighs, cut in cubes
- 1 cinnamon stick
- 2 cups of unsalted crushed tomato

- 1 1/2 cups of water
- 1 cardamom pod
- 1 cup of basmati rice
- 1/2 cup of yogurt
- 1 tsp. of ground cumin
- 1/2 tsp. of turmeric
- 2 slices of ginger
- 1 tsp. of garam masala
- 2 tsps. Of olive oil
- 1 bay leaf
- 2 cloves of garlic
- 1 onion

Instructions

- Inside a mixer, puree the onion, ginger, and garlic.
- One tbsp. oil should be heated. Cumin, garam masala, and cayenne pepper are browned with the pureed mixture.
- You need to cook, stirring frequently, for 2 mins after including the tomatoes.
- Diminish flame to low, stir in yogurt, and cook for 10 mins, stirring constantly. Remove the pot out of the flame and set it aside.
- One tbsp. oil should be included. Then chicken should be included and cooked till mildly browned.
- Stir in a few spoonsful of sauce and continue to cook till the liquid has decreased and the chicken has lost its pinkness. Inside a big-sized mixing container, mix simultaneously the cooked chicken and the sauce. Cilantro is a great inclusion.
- Cook on low flame for 5 to 10 mins. Stir once in a while.
- In a sauce pot, warm the oil. Whisk in the rice and spices and toast for a few mins. Then water needs to be included. Bring the water to the boil. Cover and cook for around 15 mins on low flame.

55. Fresh Herb Cranberry Stuffing

Preparation time nine mins Cooking Time forty-five mins
Servings six persons
Nutritional facts 143 calories Carb 21 gm Protein 4 gm Fat 8 gm Sodium 202 mg Potassium 106 mg Phosphorous 44 mg
Ingredients

- ½ cup of cranberries, dried, sweetened
- ¼ cup (1/2 stick) of unsalted butter
- ½ cup of sliced celery
- ¼ cup of giblet stock
- 2 teaspoons of poultry seasoning
- ½ tablespoon of every fresh parsley, rosemary, sage, thyme
- ½ tsp. of black pepper
- ½ cup of sliced onion
- 8 bread slices, cut into ½-inch cubes
- ½ cup of low-cholesterol egg product

Instructions

- In a nonstick frying pot, melt the butter. Onion & celery should be sautéed. Remove the pot from the flame.
- Mix the poultry seasoning, cubed bread, fresh herbs, pepper, and cranberries in a big-sized mixing container. Mix the egg product and the giblet stock inside a mixing container. Put into the bread mixture and whisk mildly to mix. To cook the stuffing, put it in the turkey's body cavity and neck.
- Cook separately for 45 mins at 350F in a baking dish sprayed using nonstick cooking spray.

56. Turkey Meatballs with Hot Sauce

Preparation time nine mins Cooking Time twenty-one mins
Servings fifteen persons
Nutritional facts 68.4 calories Carb 3.7 gm Protein 5.7 gm Fat 3.1gm Sodium 58 mg Potassium 88 mg Phosphorous 100 mg
Ingredients
- ¼ cup of minced bell pepper
- 1 lb. of lean ground turkey
- ½ cup of unseasoned bread crumbs
- ½ cup of apple jelly
- 1 tsp. of diminished sodium soy sauce
- ½ cup of coffee rich (nondairy creamer)
- ¼ cup of minced onion
- 1 egg white
- ½ tsp. of cayenne pepper
- 2 tsps. of Italian seasoning

Instructions
- Warm up your oven at 400 ⁰ F.
- Inside a big-sized mixing container, mix simultaneously all Ingredients except the jelly & cayenne pepper. Create 45 meatballs out of the mixture.
- On a baking sheet, bake meatballs for around 20 mins, or till cooked through.
- oven the jelly & cayenne for around one min, or till liquefied.
- Put meatballs in a serving dish and cover with jelly.

57. Oven Roasted Chicken and Warm Mushroom Salad with Watercress

Preparation time nine mins Cooking Time nine mins
Servings two persons
Nutritional facts 340 calories Carb 6 gm Protein 31 gm Fat 21 gm Sodium 77 mg Potassium 420 mg Phosphorous 251 mg
Ingredients
- 2 tbsps. of balsamic vinegar
- Black peppercorns
- 1/2 tsp. of thyme
- 4 tbsps. of olive oil
- 1 cup of assorted wild mushrooms
- 4 cups of mixed greens (comprising the watercress)
- Half cup of shallots

Instructions
- Black pepper and thyme are used to season the chicken.
- Drizzle with olive oil.
- Warm up your oven at 350°F and bake till the inside is no longer pink.

- In a griddle, brown mushrooms as well as shallots in olive oil. Finish with balsamic vinegar and season using fresh thyme.
- Slice the chicken and serve it over a bed of greens with warm mushrooms.

58. Spicy Chicken Penne

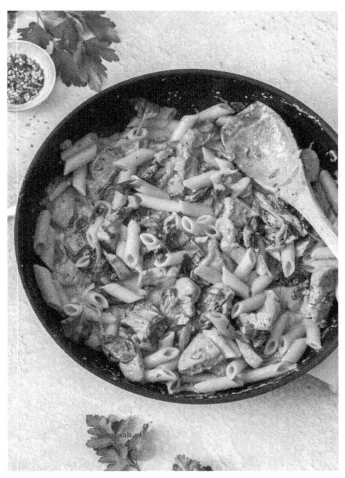

Preparation time five mins Cooking Time nine mins
Servings four persons
Nutritional facts 392 calories Carb 39 gm Protein 34 gm Fat 10 gm Sodium 137 mg Potassium 639 mg
Phosphorous 335 mg
Ingredients
- 2 tablespoons of olive oil, divided
- 2 cups of dried penne pasta
- 1 lb. of chicken breast (raw), cut into 3"" x 1"" inch strips
- ¼ to ½ teaspoon of red pepper flakes, crushed
- 2 tbsps. of parmesan cheese
- 3 green onions, cut into half inch pieces
- 24 grape cherry or cherry tomatoes
- 2 cloves of garlic, minced
- ¼ cup of sliced fresh basil
Instructions
- Cook pasta as per the package directions inside a big-sized pot of boiling water without the salt.
- Drain the pasta, reserving 1/2 cup of the cooking water.

- One tablespoon olive oil should be heated in a big-sized nonstick griddle on moderate high flame.
- Cook for around 2 to 3 mins after including the chicken strips.
- Diminish the flame to moderate & put in the rest of the one tablespoon of oil.
- Whisk in the red pepper flakes, tomatoes, and garlic.
- Cook for around 3 to 4 mins, or till tomatoes burst & chicken is fully cooked.
- Cook for one min after including cooked penne and green onions to the pot.
- Mix parmesan cheese and basil inside a mixing container. To achieve the desired consistency, include the saved pasta cooking liquid.

59. Moroccan Chicken

Preparation time one day Cooking Time forty mins
Servings six persons
Nutritional facts 196 calories Carb 16 gm Protein 26 gm Fat 3 gm Sodium 79 mg Potassium 305 mg Phosphorous 218 mg
Ingredients

- 2 tablespoons of lemon juice
- 1/3 cup of honey
- ½ teaspoon of cayenne pepper
- ½ teaspoon of lemon zest
- ¼ teaspoon of black pepper
- ¼ teaspoon of onion powder
- 1 teaspoon of paprika
- ¼ teaspoon of nutmeg
- 1 teaspoon of sesame oil
- 3 cloves of garlic—crushed
- ½ teaspoon of ground cumin
- 6 chicken breasts or thighs—bone in, no skin
- ¼ teaspoon of cinnamon

Instructions

- Mix the Ingredients and marinate the chicken.
- Refrigerate for one to 24 hrs, flipping a few times as needed.
- Then use foil to line a baking sheet. Put the chicken, bone-side down, on foil. Put the rest of the marinade on top.
- Warm up your oven at 400°F and bake for 30–40 mins, or till thoroughly cooked.

60. Stir Fry Rice Noodles with Chicken and Basil

Preparation time fourteen mins Cooking Time five mins
Servings six persons
Nutritional facts 292 calories Carb 35 gm Protein 19 gm Fat 8 gm Sodium 131 mg Potassium 320 mg Phosphorous 234 mg
Ingredients

- 1 tbsp. of garlic, minced
- 8 oz. of rice noodles
- 2 tbsps. of cilantro, sliced
- 1 tbsp. of sesame oil
- 3 big skinless chicken breasts, sliced finely
- 2 eggs, beaten

- 6 sliced green onions
- 4 tbsps. of fresh basil, sliced
- juice of two limes
- 1 tbsp. of vegetable oil
- red chilies (optional)
- 1 tbsp. of ginger, minced

Instructions

- Soak for around ten mins in warm water.
- Drain the water and set it aside.
- In a frying pot or wok, warm the oil.
- Garlic, ginger, & chicken should be stir-fried till the chicken is cooked through.
- Cook for a few mins more after including the green onions and noodles to the pot/wok.
- Stir in the eggs as well as lime juice till the eggs are thoroughly mixed.
- Include the basil and cilantro at the end.
- Serve right away.

61. Jerk Chicken Wings

Preparation time three mins Cooking Time thirty-five mins
Servings six persons
Nutritional facts 382.4 calories Carb 0.4 gm Protein 27.4 gm Fat 29.5 gm Sodium 84 mg Potassium 194.6 mg Phosphorous 155 mg
Ingredients

- 1/3 tsp. of cayenne pepper
- 18 chicken wings
- One teaspoon of dry thyme
- Half tsp. of cinnamon
- One teaspoon of all spice
- Quarter cup of vegetable oil

Instructions

- The oven should be warmed up to 450 F.
- Mix dry spices with vegetable oil to create the JERK sauce.
- Baste chicken wings using sauce.
- Then it should be baked for around 30-35 mins.

Chapter 3: Salads and Sandwiches

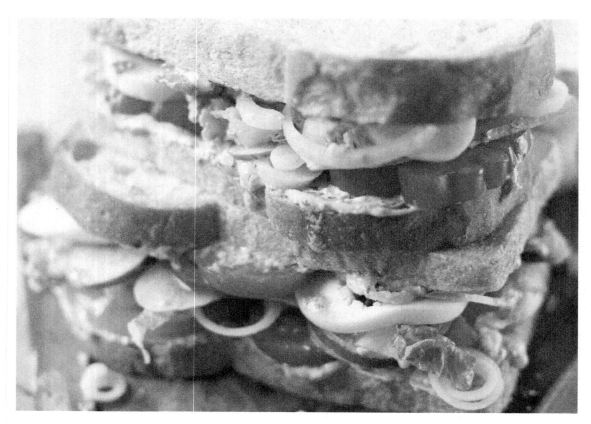

This chapter is dedicated to renal-friendly salads and sandwiches recipes.

1. Chickpea Sunflower Sandwich

Preparation time twenty mins Cooking Time zero mins
Servings four persons
Nutritional facts 388 calories Carb 52.8 gm Protein 15.7 gm Fat 13.5 gm Sodium 570.2 mg Potassium 378.6 mg Phosphorous 317.3 mg
Ingredients

- 2 tablespoons of fresh dill
- 1/4 cup of prepared hummus
- Two teaspoons of fresh dill
- 1/4 cup of roasted sunflower seeds
- 3 tablespoons of vegan mayonnaise or tahini
- A half teaspoon of Dijon or spicy mustard
- One 15-ounces can of chickpeas, drained & washed
- A half lemon, juiced (around 1 tablespoon)
- 1 tablespoon of maple syrup
- 1/4 cup of red onion, sliced
- One pinch of pepper
- 8 slices of low sodium whole wheat bread
- 2 cloves of garlic, minced
- water as needed to thin sauce
- Sliced avocado, onion, lettuce, tomato

Instructions

- Mix lemon, dill, hummus, as well as minced garlic inside a container to create the garlic herb sauce.
- Then it should be put away.
- Mix the dill, red onion, and pepper inside a big-sized mixing container.
- Toast the bread in a little oil or vegan butter.
- Fill four slices of bread with a qtr. of your chickpea & sunflower seed filling. Whisk in the garlic herb sauce as well as any additional seasonings. Put the rest of the four slices of bread on top.

2. Bourbon-Glazed Skirt Steak

Preparation time seventeen mins Cooking Time forty-eight mins
Servings six persons
Nutritional facts 409 calories Carb 8 gm Protein 24 gm Fat 22 gm Sodium 152 mg Potassium 283 mg Phosphorous 171mg
Ingredients

- Bourbon Glaze:
- 1 tablespoon of black pepper
- 2 tablespoons of Dijon mustard
- Skirt Steak:
- ¼ cup of dark brown sugar
- 2 tablespoons of grape seed oil
- A half teaspoon of smoked paprika
- ½ teaspoon of dried oregano
- 1 teaspoon of black pepper
- 3 tablespoons of unsalted butter, cubed and chilled
- 2 pounds of skirt steak
- A quarter cup of diced shallots
- 1 cup of bourbon
- One tablespoon of red wine vinegar

Instructions

- Brown shallots in 1 tbsp. butter in a small-sized saucepot over moderate-high flame.
- Diminish the flame to lower, remove the pot from the flame, and include the bourbon prior to returning the saucepot to the flame.
- Cook for ten to 15 mins, or when the liquid has been diminished by one-third.
- Stir in the mustard, brown sugar, & black pepper till the mixture is bubbly.
- Flip off the flame as well as mix in the rest of the two tablespoons of cubed, cold butter till thoroughly mixed.
- In a sealable storage bag that is gallon-size, mix the Ingredients, then include the steaks & then shake well.
- Give the steaks for around 30 to 45 mins to marinate inside the bag at room temperature.
- Remove the steaks from the bag and grill for approximately 20 mins on every side and then put away for around ten mins to rest.
- Slice the dish and drizzle it with sauce, or leave it whole and glaze it, and broil for around 4 to 6 mins, or till desired appearance is achieved.

3. Crunchy Apple-Maple Snack Mix

Preparation time ten mins Cooking Time twenty-five mins
Servings 26 persons
Nutritional facts 144 calories Carb 26.7 gm Protein 1.5 gm Fat 4.1 gm Sodium 89.6 mg Potassium 61.8 mg Phosphorous 37.3 mg
Ingredients

- 1/3 cup of Brown Sugar
- 3 cups of Graham Cereal
- 10 oz. (1 box) of Teddy Grahams snack cookies
- 3 oz. of Dried Apples
- 6 oz. of Pretzels
- 1/2 cup of Unsalted Butter
- 5 oz. of Dried Cranberries
- 1/4 cup of Honey
- 5 cups of Rice Chex
- Two cups of Apple Straws
- 1/4 cup of Maple Syrup

Instructions

- Inside a big-sized mixing container, mix Rice Chex, graham cereal, Apple Straws (optional), Teddy Grahams and pretzels.
- Inside a small-sized saucepot, melt the butter; put the honey, brown sugar, and maple syrup. Cook, stirring constantly, till the sugar has dissolved.
- Put over the cereal mixture and whisk well to coat all of the pieces.
- Warm up your oven at 325 º F.
- Arrange 3 jelly roll pots on a baking sheet lined using aluminum foil and sprayed using cooking spray.
- Using a spoon, evenly distribute the cereal mixture between the pots. Warm up your oven at 325°F and bake for 20 mins, stirring halfway through.
- Mix cranberries and Apple Chips inside a mixing container; divide evenly among pots and stir to mix.
- Bake for an additional 5 mins, then cool completely prior to storing in an sealed container.

4. Pimento Cream Cheese Sandwiches

Preparation time ten mins Cooking Time zero mins
Servings two persons
Nutritional facts 304 calories Carb 32 gm Protein 8 gm Fat 16 gm Sodium 411 mg Potassium 137 mg Phosphorous 101 mg
Ingredients

- 1/8 teaspoon of pepper
- A half cup of whipped cream cheese
- 1/2 teaspoon of sugar
- One tablespoon of tinned pimento
- Four slices of bread

Instructions

- Pimento should be diced. Mix the whipped cream cheese, sugar, pimento, and pepper inside a small-sized mixing container.
- To create sandwiches, spread 1/4 cup of the mixture on your preferred bread.

5. Pressed Vegetarian Picnic Sandwich

Preparation time ten mins Cooking Time thirty-seven mins
Servings four persons
Nutritional facts 466 calories Carb 78.1 gm Protein 20.5 gm Fat 8.8 gm Sodium 851.7 mg Potassium 560 mg Phosphorous 244.1 mg
Ingredients

- 1 Tbsp. of green olives

- 2–9" French baguettes
- 1 Tbsp. of Kalamata olives
- A half cup of roasted red pepper, sliced
- 1 Tbsp. of black olives, low sodium
- 1/4 cup of Olive Oil
- 1 Tbsp. of Fresh Parsley, coarsely sliced
- 3 eggs, hard boiled and sliced
- 1 cup of green beans, trimmed
- 1 Tbsp. of Fresh Basil
- A half tsp. of Dijon Mustard
- 1 moderate eggplant, sliced into disks
- 1 1/2 tsp. of coarsely sliced Shallots
- A half tsp. of Sugar
- 1 Tbsp. of low sodium black olives

Instructions

- To create sandwiches, follow these steps: Warm up your oven at 350 º F. Coat baking sheet using nonstick cooking spray. Coat a baking sheet using cooking spray and arrange eggplant slices in a single layer. If desired, season using pepper. Bake for 20 mins, flipping once, or till browned and tender.
- Meanwhile, cook green beans till tender in a big-sized pot of boiling water (or steam). Drain and wash thoroughly with cold water. Using paper towels thoroughly dry the area.
- To create the vinaigrette, mix simultaneously all of the Ingredients inside a mixer and blend till smooth. Inside a mixer or food processor, mix the shallots, mustard (optional), olive oil, basil, parsley, vinegar, and sugar till smooth.
- Remove the most of the tender white bread from the baguette halves' centers. Then in the hollow lower part half spread the tapenade. Brush with the vinaigrette. Put green beans on top of tapenade and press down firmly. Top with egg slices, red pepper slices, and eggplant slices.
- Brush the inside of the baguette top with vinaigrette and put eggplant slices on top. Sandwiches should be pressed simultaneously and tied with twine or tightly wrapped in wax paper or plastic wrap. Chill for 1 to 4 hrs. With a serrated knife, cut into 4 Servings as well as serve with any rest of the vinaigrette.

6. Walnut and Kidney Bean Spread (Lobio)

Preparation time ten mins Cooking Time ten mins
Servings ten persons
Nutritional facts 102 calories Carb 14.6 gm Protein 3.5 gm Fat 2.9 gm Sodium 291.9 mg Potassium 213 mg Phosphorous 185 mg
Ingredients

- Two 15-ounce cans of kidney beans washed & drained
- 1/3 cup of sliced walnuts
- Two tablespoons of red wine vinegar
- Generous grating black pepper
- 2-3 tablespoons of vegetable broth
- Two cloves of garlic
- 1/4 teaspoon of salt or as required
- 1/8 teaspoon of cayenne pepper or as required
- 3 tablespoons of finely sliced green onions
- Three tablespoons of minced parsley

Instructions

- In a food processor, mix the walnuts & garlic and process till finely sliced, stopping the machine and scraping down the sides as needed. Process the vinegar, 2 tbsps. broth, cayenne, salt, and black pepper till a chunky paste forms. If necessary, include more broth.
- Insert the well-drained beans to the processor and pulse 6–8 times, just long enough to crush but not puree the beans.
- Scrape half of the parsley as well as green onions into a big-sized container and stir to mix. The rest should be sprinkled on top. To allow flavors to blend, cover and chill for around an hr. Taste for seasoning and include more vinegar, pepper, or salt as needed.

7. Chicken 'n' Grape Salad Sandwich

Preparation time ten mins Cooking Time ten mins
Servings six persons
Nutritional facts 145 calories Carb 11 gm Protein 8 gm Fat 8 gm Sodium 100 mg Potassium 165 mg Phosphorous 245 mg
Ingredients

- A quarter cup of onion, diced
- 1 cup of cooked chicken, sliced
- A one third cup of mayonnaise
- ½ cup of sliced green pepper
- A half cup of celery, diced
- 1 cup of grapes, sliced

Instructions

- Mix the chicken, green pepper, celery, and onion inside a mixing container.
- Mix the sliced grapes as well as mayonnaise inside a mixing container.
- Gently mix the Ingredients.
- On a piece of bread, a tortilla, a roll, or a pita, spread the chicken and grape mixture.
- Serve with a side of crisp lettuce or other greens.
- Serve with fruit, either fresh or tinned.

8. Honey-Maple Mix

Preparation time ten mins Cooking Time thirty mins
Servings six persons
Nutritional facts 262 calories Carb 47 gm Protein 3 gm Fat 9 gm Sodium 178 mg Potassium 84 mg Phosphorous 66 mg
Ingredients

- 5 cups of Rice Chex cereal
- 3 cups of Golden Grahams cereal
- 10 ounces of Cinnamon Teddy Grahams snack cookies
- 1/4 cup of honey
- A quarter cup of maple syrup
- 3 ounces of Crispy Granny Smith Apple Chips
- 1/3 cup of dark brown sugar
- A half cup of unsalted butter
- 5 ounces of dried cranberries, sweetened
- 6 ounces of Pretzel Crisps

Instructions

- Inside a big-sized mixing container, mix Golden Grahams, Teddy Grahams, Rice Chex, and pretzels.
- Inside a small-sized saucepot, melt the butter; put the honey, brown sugar, and maple syrup. Cook, stirring constantly, till the sugar has dissolved.

- Put over the cereal mixture and whisk well to coat all of the pieces.
- Warm up your oven at 325 º F.
- Arrange 3 jelly roll pots on a baking sheet lined using aluminum foil and sprayed using cooking spray. This can be done in three batches. Using a spoon, evenly distribute the cereal mixture between the pots. Warm up your oven at 325°F and bake for 20 mins, stirring halfway through.
- Mix cranberries and Apple Chips inside a mixing container; divide equally among pots and stir to mix.
- Bake for an additional 5 mins, then cool completely prior to storing in an sealed container.

9. Low Sodium Guacamole

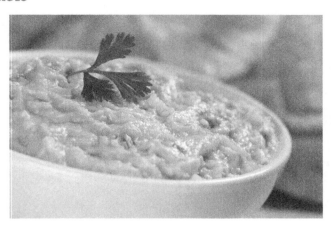

Preparation time five mins Cooking Time zero mins
Servings six persons
Nutritional facts 44 calories Carb 4 gm Protein 1 gm Fat 4 gm Sodium 29 mg Potassium 149 mg
Phosphorous 19 mg
Ingredients
- 1 pinch of salt
- A quarter cup of onion minced
- 1 big avocado tender
- 2 cloves of garlic minced
- One lime juiced
- 1 jalapeno minced
- A quarter cup of fresh cilantro sliced

Instructions
- Mix avocado and lime juice inside a container.
- Then it is to be mashed with a fork to desired consistency.
- Then put in the rest of the Ingredients. Mix well and enjoy.

10. Low Oxalate Granola

Preparation time ten mins Cooking Time twenty-five mins
Servings twelve persons
Nutritional facts 155 calories Carb 80 gm Protein 4 gm Fat 7 gm Sodium 45 mg Potassium 63 mg
Phosphorous 35 mg
Ingredients
- A quarter teaspoon of kosher salt
- 1.25 teaspoon of vanilla extract
- A half cup of unsalted sunflower seeds
- 3 cups of rolled old fashioned oats (use gluten-free if you are gluten intolerant)
- 1.5 teaspoon of ground cinnamon

- Two tablespoons of vegetable oil
- 1/2 cup of unsalted pistachios
- A half cup of no sugar included dried cranberries
- 2 Tablespoons of sugar-free pancake syrup

Instructions

- Warm up your oven at 325 º F.
- Mix dried cranberries, oats, oil, sunflower seeds, pistachios, vanilla extract, and pancake syrup inside a big-sized mixing container. With a spoon, mix everything simultaneously till it's evenly mixed.
- Mix the cinnamon and salt in a mixing dish.
- Spray your baking sheet using cooking spray and line it with parchment paper.
- Create sure the granola is evenly distributed on the baking sheet.
- Bake for ten min, then stir and continue baking for another 5 mins, or till golden brown.
- Take the food out of the oven & then let it cool prior to serving.

11. Sweet & Nutty Protein Bars

Preparation time fifteen mins Cooking Time one hr twenty mins
Servings twelve persons
Nutritional facts 283 calories Carb 39 gm Protein 7 gm Fat 13 gm Sodium 49 mg Potassium 258 mg Phosphorous 177 mg
Ingredients

- A half cup of peanut butter
- 2½ cups of rolled oats, toasted
- 1 cup of dried blueberries, cherries or Craisins
- A half cup of almonds
- ½ cup of flaxseeds
- A half cup of honey

Instructions

- Put rolled oats on a baking sheet and toast for ten mins or till golden brown in a 350° F oven.
- Mix simultaneously all Ingredients inside a big-sized mixing container and stir till thoroughly mixed.
- In a mildly greased 9" x 9" pot, press the protein mixture down. Wrap in plastic wrap and chill for around sixty mins or overnight.
- Serve protein bars after being cut into desired squares.

12. Clean Eating Egg Salad Sandwich Recipe

Preparation time thirteen mins Cooking Time zero mins
Servings two persons
Nutritional facts 295 calories Carb 23 gm Protein 16 gm Fat 14 gm
Sodium 377 mg Potassium 242 mg Phosphorous 168 mg
Ingredients

- Half small avocado
- Four slices of whole grain bread (no sugar included)
- 3 big eggs (hard boiled, peeled & sliced)
- 1 tbsp. of mayonnaise
- One small tomato (sliced or sliced fine)

Instructions

- Smash the avocado with a fork inside a moderate-sized mixing container.
- Mix the rest of the Ingredients as well as blend well till it achieves the consistency of guacamole.

- Put the filling in the middle of two slices of bread.
- If you want, you can include to your sandwich lettuce or cucumber slices.

13. Rice Roti Upma | Rice Bhakri Poha | Kottu Pathiri

Preparation time ten mins Cooking Time ten mins
Servings two persons
Nutritional facts 167 calories Carb 34 gm Protein 3 gm Fat 2 gm Sodium 5 mg Potassium 75 mg
Phosphorous 63 mg
Ingredients

- 1/4 tsp. of Finely Sliced Green Chili
- A quarter tsp. of Mustard Seeds
- 4 Rice Rotis
- Salt as required
- 1/2 tsp. of Oil
- 1/4 tsp. of Cumin Seeds
- 1/8 tsp. of Turmeric
- A quarter cup of Finely Sliced Onion
- A Few Curry Leaves

Instructions

- The 4 x 7" rice rotis are to be cut into 1/2" pieces. You can grind it to a fine powder. Use 6 rotis if you're going to create a coarse powder.
- Warm ½ teaspoon oil in a kadhai.
- Stir in 1/2 teaspoon mustard seeds and wait for them to splutter.
- Then insert half tsp finely sliced green chilies and 1/2 tsp. of cumin seeds. For a few secs, stir-fry.
- Stir-fry for another few secs with 4 to 6 curry leaves.
- Stir in a quarter cup finely sliced onions and cook till they are transparent.
- Mix in a pinch of salt and 1/8 teaspoon of turmeric.
- Mix in the rice roti pieces thoroughly.
- Flip the flame off.
- Then it is to be sprinkled with one or two tsp water, and mixed thoroughly.
- Cover and put away for 5 mins.
- Rice Roti Upma should be served with Dahi on the side.

Chapter 4: Renal-Friendly Dinner Recipes

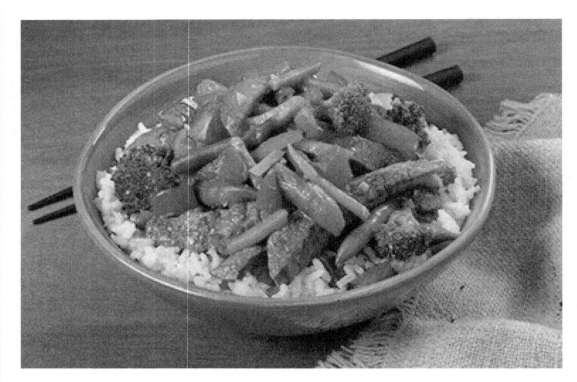

It is night time and here are the most nutritious and renal-friendly dinner recipes for you.

1. Plant-Based Meal Prep Burrito Container

Preparation time fifteen mins Cooking Time fifteen mins
Servings six persons
Nutritional facts 423 calories Carb 60 gm Protein 9 gm Fat 17 gm Sodium 529 mg Potassium 456 mg Phosphorous 268 mg
Ingredients

- 1 teaspoon of smoked paprika
- One and a half cups of white rice dry and uncooked
- 1 teaspoon every of ground cumin, smoked paprika chili powder, & garlic powder
- 1 lime juiced, as required
- 2 moderate red bell peppers, seeds discarded and sliced
- 1 cup of corn
- Quarter teaspoon of chili powder
- 1 teaspoon of adobo sauce
- 2 moderate sliced onions
- ¼ cup of avocado oil
- 3 cups of water or per package directions
- ¼ cup of coconut milk yogurt
- ¼ teaspoon of salt as required
- Optional Seasonings: sliced romaine lettuce, a squeeze of lime juice, cubed avocado, diced tomatoes or salsa, sliced cilantro
- Quarter cup of vegan mayonnaise
- 2 cups of tinned black beans, drained & washed

Instructions

- Three cups of water should be used to cook the rice in a rice cooker or pot, or as directed on the package.
- Inside a small-sized container, mix the yogurt, chili powder, vegan mayonnaise, smoked paprika, lime juice, and adobo sauce. If necessary, include water to change the consistency.
- Then, put a big griddle over moderate flame and include avocado oil. Include the pepper & onion slices; cook, including just a little water if required to avoid burning, cook the veggies for seven to ten mins, stirring occasionally, till they are tender and tender. After that, include the seasonings, black beans, and corn. Cook for an extra two to three mins, or till the corn is warmed through but still has some crunch.
- The cooked rice should now be divided among four containers or containers. After that, include the fajita mixture to the rice and include any additional seasonings. Just prior to serving, drizzle the chipotle dressing.

2. Low Sodium Sloppy Joes

Preparation time ten mins Cooking Time thirty mins
Servings six persons
Nutritional facts 148 calories Carb 10 gm Protein 19 gm Fat 4 gm Sodium 238 mg Potassium 437 mg Phosphorous 169 mg
Ingredients

- 1/8 tsp. of crushed red pepper flakes
- One and a quarter pounds of ground sirloin
- 5 tbsps. of ketchup
- 2 tbsps. of chili powder
- 1/3 cup of water
- 2 tsps. of brown sugar
- 1/2 big onion diced
- 2 tbsps. of low sodium tomato paste
- 1/2 tsps. of ground mustard
- 3 cloves of garlic minced
- 1/2 big green bell pepper diced
- 2 tbsps. of apple cider vinegar

Instructions

- The ground sirloin should be browned in a big sauté pot.
- Once the tomato paste has a deep red hue, include it and simmer it for one to two mins. Include the garlic, green pepper, and onion. Around three to five mins of cooking are needed to mildly tendered the vegetables.
- Then the rest of the Ingredients should be mixed well. Cook for 10-15 mins with a cover.

3. Kidney Friendly Vegan Mayo

Preparation and Cooking Time ten mins
Servings 25 Servings
Nutritional facts 82 calories Carb 1 gm Protein 1 gm Fat 9 gm Sodium 4 mg Potassium 7 mg Phosphorous 2 mg
Ingredients

- One and a half tbsps. of lemon juice or cider/white vinegar
- Half cup of unsweetened soy milk
- 1 cup of vegetable oil

- Half a teaspoon of mustard powder
- 1 tsp. of Dijon mustard

Instructions

- A container appropriate for an immersion mixer should be used to mix the lemon juice, mustard powder, and unsweetened soy milk.
- Include a drop of oil at a time while blending to create an emulsion. Put a steady stream of oil very slowly once the mixture has emulsified.
- Include Dijon mustard.

4. Egg Fried Rice

Preparation time ten mins
Servings six persons
Nutritional facts 137 calories Carb 21 gm Protein 5 gm Fat 4 gm Sodium 38 mg Potassium 89 mg Phosphorous 67 mg
Ingredients

- 1 tablespoon of canola oil
- 2 teaspoons of dark sesame oil
- 1 cup of frozen peas, thawed
- 1 cup of bean sprouts
- ¼ teaspoon of ground black pepper
- 4 cups of cooked rice, cold
- ⅓ cup of green onions, sliced
- 2 eggs
- 2 egg whites

Instructions

- Inside a small-sized container, mix the egg whites, sesame oil, and eggs. Stir thoroughly and reserve.
- Big-sized nonstick griddle with canola oil should be heated to moderate-high flame.
- Once finished, stir-fry the egg mixture in.
- Include green onions with the bean sprouts. It should be stir-fried for two mins.
- Now include rice and peas. Stir-fry till everything is well hot.
- Serve right away after sprinkling black pepper.

5. Kidney Friendly Honey Mustard Chicken

Preparation time fifteen mins Cooking Time twenty-five mins
Servings four persons
Nutritional facts 240.23 calories Carb 24.9 gm Protein 30.03 gm Fat 2.69 gm Sodium 246.93 mg Potassium 231.1 mg Phosphorous 165.2 mg
Ingredients

- Two cups of Mushrooms, raw
- One lb. of Boneless & Skinless Chicken Breast Portions
- One tsp. of Seasoned pepper, salt free
- 12 ounces of Broccoli cuts
- ¾ cup of honey mustard sauce

Instructions

- Remove the vegetables from the water after washing and set them aside to dry.
- Warm up a nonstick griddle over moderate-high flame.

- Cut the chicken breasts into bite-size pieces and cook them in a sauté pot till light brown.
- Continue to cook the chicken pieces in the pot with the broccoli cuts and pepper till they are tender crisp. Cook till the mushrooms are light brown in color.
- Diminish to a low flame setting and stir in the mustard sauce and honey. Simmer for 10-15 min with the lid on the pot.
- Put 1/2 cup of the mixture on a serving plate and serve right away. Save leftovers for around three days in the fridge.

6. Easy Dutch Oven Rustic Bread

Preparation time five mins Cooking Time one hr forty mins
Servings fourteen persons
Nutritional facts 157 calories Carb 33 gm Protein 4 gm Fat 0 gm Sodium 201 mg Potassium 213 mg Phosphorous 123 mg
Ingredients

- 4.5 cups of All Purpose Flour
- Two tsps. of Active Dry Yeast
- Two cups of Lukewarm Water, around 110 ^{0}
- 2 Tbsps. of Honey
- One Tbsp. of Kosher Salt

Instructions

- Mix honey, yeast, and water inside your stand mixer container.
- Stir a little more to ensure that the honey dissolves.
- Permit to sit for around ten mins, or till it begins to foam.
- Mix the flour as well as salt simultaneously inside a separate container.
- Include the dough attachment to the mixer once the yeast is ready.
- Begin including the flour mixture to the mixer on low speed with a 1 cup measuring scoop.
- Continue in this manner, allowing the flour to absorb the liquid prior to including more.
- A rubber spoon may be required to scrape the sides of the mixer.
- It's fine if the mixture is sticky.
- After you've included all of the flour as well as the mixture is starting to come simultaneously, increase the speed of the mixer low to moderate.
- Allow the mixer to knead the dough till it forms a ball.
- It could take around ten mins for this to happen, but it will.
- You'll notice that the dough is no longer sticking to the sides of the container...this is where the magic happens.
- Stop, remove the hook, and cover the mixing container using plastic wrap, permitting the dough to rest for 30-40 mins in a draft-free area of your kitchen.
- It will rise during this time.
- Put the Dutch oven (uncovered) in the oven and warm up to 400 ^{0} after 20 mins.
- Remove the Dutch oven from the oven with care and spray it with nonstick spray.
- Remove the plastic wrap from the dough and flour the top.
- A small amount of flour should be sprinkled over the top of the dough. Put the Dutch oven in the oven, covered.
- Cover the bread and bake it for thirty mins.
- Remove the lid out of the Dutch oven and bake it for an additional 10-15 mins, or till it begins to brown.

- Carefully take the Dutch oven out of the oven, allowing it to cool completely inside it prior to removing it.
- Your bread has been baked.
- Cut into slices and eat.
- Now you'll transfer the dough to the Dutch oven, which has been warmed up.
- A small amount of flour should be sprinkled over the top of the dough.

7. French Canadian Shepherd's Pie – Pate Chinois

Preparation time fifteen mins Cooking Time one hr zero mins
Servings six persons
Nutritional facts 230 calories Carb 22 gm Protein 19 gm Fat 7 gm Sodium 82 mg Potassium 665 mg Phosphorous 219 mg
Ingredients

- A half cup of unsweetened original almond milk
- 1 lb. of peeled and diced potatoes
- 1 sliced yellow onion
- One lb. of lean ground beef
- Two cups of unsalted whole kernel corn
- One tbsp. of olive oil

Instructions

- Warm up your oven at 350 º F (175 º Celsius).
- In a saucepot, boil the diced potatoes for around ten mins, or till they can be pierced using a fork easily. If you're concerned around your potassium intake, consider boiling the potatoes twice.
- Cook the sliced onion in olive oil till golden in a pot during this time.
- Cook till the ground beef is mildly browned and crisp in the pot. While cooking, break up the meat finely in the pot using a wooden spoon.
- When the potatoes are done boiling, drain them and put them inside a container.
- Put in the milk as well as mash the potatoes with a fork or a masher till they are smooth. Include more milk if it isn't smooth enough. When you're ready, set it aside.
- Put the meat on the lower part of an 8" x 8" square dish.
- Over the meat, spread a uniform layer of whole kernel corn.
- Create a layer of mashed potatoes that is uniform in thickness.
- Warm up your oven at 350°F and bake the dish for 30 mins, just till the mashed potato layer is golden.
- Warm up your oven at 500°F (260°C) and broil for 2-3 mins. Remove from the oven when the top is golden and let it cool prior to serving.

8. Smoothie Recipe (Low Potassium Version)

Preparation time five mins Cooking Time zero mins
Servings two persons
Nutritional facts 265.76 calories Carb 36.91 gm Protein 14.27 gm Fat 8.68 gm Sodium 108.41 mg Potassium 96.28mg Phosphorous 120.6 mg
Ingredients

- 2 scoops of Dietician approved protein powder
- 1 cup of fresh berries
- 2/3 cup of ice
- A half cup of frozen pineapple
- One cup of rice milk
- Two to three tablespoons of hemp hearts or chia seeds

Instructions

- Mix all of the components inside the mixer.
- You can put in more ice or liquid to achieve required consistency.

9. Slow-Cooked Lemon Chicken

Preparation time 30 mins Cooking Time, 5 hrs 35 mins
Servings 4 persons
Nutritional facts 197 calories Carb 1 gm Protein 26 gm Fat 9 gm Sodium 57 mg Potassium 412 mg Phosphorous 251 mg
Ingredients
- Two cloves of garlic, minced
- 1 teaspoon of dried oregano
- ¼ cup of chicken broth, low sodium
- A quarter teaspoon of ground black pepper
- 2 tablespoons of butter, unsalted
- A quarter cup of water
- One pound of chicken breast, boneless, & skinless
- 1 tablespoon of lemon juice
- One tsp. of fresh basil, sliced

Instructions
- Inside a small-sized container, mix oregano with black pepper. The chicken should be rubbed on the mixture.
- Inside a moderate-sized griddle, melt butter on moderate flame. Move the chicken to the slow cooker after browning it in the dissolved butter.
- In a griddle, mix the chicken broth, lemon juice, water, and garlic. To get the browned bits off the lower part of the griddle, bring it to boil. Put the sauce over the chicken.
- Cover and cook on high for two and a half hrs or low for five hrs in a slow cooker.
- Whisk in the basil and baste the chicken. Cook for an additional 15 to 30 mins on high, or till chicken is tender.

10. Roasted Chicken Breasts

Preparation time five mins Cooking Time thirty-five mins
Servings four persons
Nutritional facts 170 calories Carb 3 gm Protein 24 gm Fat 6 gm Sodium 60 mg Potassium 178 mg Phosphorous 116 mg
Ingredients
- One and a half teaspoons of paprika
- 1 nonstick cooking spray
- Four chicken breasts (4-ounces every, skinless, & boneless)
- A half tsp. of black pepper
- lemon juice 1/4 cup
- One tbsp. of olive oil
- garlic (minced) 2 tbsps.
- 1 tsp. of salt (optional)

Instructions
- Warm up your oven at 350 º F. Using cooking spray, coat a baking sheet.
- On a baking sheet, arrange the chicken breasts.
- Mix salt, pepper, lemon juice, olive oil, and garlic inside a small-sized container and whisk to mix.
- Brush or put the lemon juice mixture evenly over every chicken breast.

- Sprinkle paprika evenly over every chicken breast and bake for 35 mins, or till the chicken's internal temperature reaches 165 ⁰ F.
- Allow the chicken breasts to rest for 10-15 mins, covered in foil, prior to actually slicing or serving.

11. Chicken, Red Pepper, Spinach and White Bean Pizza

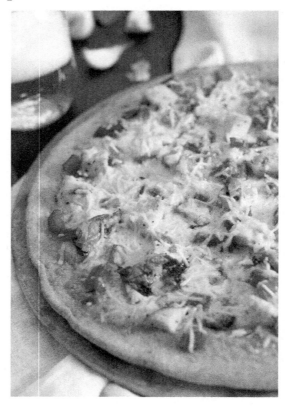

Preparation time ten mins Cooking Time twelve mins
Servings eight persons
Nutritional facts 204 calories Carb 21 gm Protein 14 gm Fat 21 gm Sodium 362 mg Potassium 264 mg Phosphorous 179 mg
Ingredients
- One cup of sliced cooked chicken breast
- One (12-inch) thin pizza crust
- 2 cups of sliced baby spinach
- One cup of shredded part-skim mozzarella cheese
- A half cup of sliced red onion
- 2 teaspoons of olive oil
- One moderate cored and finely sliced red bell pepper
- 1 teaspoon of dried oregano leaves
- One teaspoon of minced garlic
- A half cup of white navy beans, drained & washed

Instructions
- Warm up your oven at 425 ⁰ F. Using oil, coat the crust.
- Cook red pepper and onion inside a big-sized nonstick griddle coated using nonstick cooking spray for around 5 mins, or till crisp tender. Stir in the garlic, spinach, and oregano till the spinach has wilted.

- Distribute the spinach mixture evenly over the crust and top with the rest of the Ingredients. It should be baked for 8–10 mins in the oven, or till the crust is light brown and the cheese is dissolved.

12. Beef Barley Soup

Preparation time twelve mins Cooking Time one hr forty-three mins
Servings ten persons
Nutritional facts 270 calories Carb 22 gm Protein 23 gm Fat 2 gm Sodium 105 mg Potassium 675 mg Phosphorous 250 mg
Ingredients
- 1/4 cup of vegetable oil, divided
- 1/2 teaspoon of black pepper
- 1 frozen package (16 ounces) of vegetables
- 2 potatoes, soaked & diced
- 3 cups of water
- 2 carrots, diced
- 1/4 teaspoon of dried thyme
- 1 can (14.5 ounces) of chicken broth, low sodium
- 1/2 cup of barley
- 2 lbs. of beef stew meat, diced one inch cubes
- 1/2 teaspoon of garlic, minced
- 1 cup of sliced onion
- 1/2 cup of sliced mushrooms

Instructions
- First, season beef using pepper.
- Then two tbsps. oil is to be included to stew pot and sauté for five mins.
- Two more tablespoons of oil should be included with include onions, carrots and mushrooms.
- Sauté for another five mins and stir frequently.
- Garlic and thyme are to be included. Then sauté for 3 mins.
- Then chicken broth and water are included to pot.
- Then mixed vegetables, potatoes and barley are included.
- Keep stirring and bring to boil.
- It should be covered and diminish the flame.
- Simmer for sixty to ninety mins.

13. Beef or Chicken Enchiladas

Preparation time eight mins Cooking Time twenty-four mins
Servings six persons
Nutritional facts 235 calories Carb 30 gm Protein 13 gm Fat 7 gm Sodium 201 mg Potassium 222 mg Phosphorous 146 mg
Ingredients
- 12 corn tortillas
- 1 pound of lean ground beef or chicken
- 1/2 teaspoon of black pepper
- 1 can of enchilada sauce
- 1 teaspoon of cumin
- 1/2 cup of sliced onion
- 1 sliced garlic clove

Instructions
- Warm up your oven at 375 º F.

- In a frying pot, brown the meat.
- Mix the onion, cumin, garlic, & pepper inside a mixing container. Continue to cook. Stir constantly till the onions are tender.
- In a separate griddle, flame a small quantity of oil and fry tortillas.
- Every tortilla should be dipped in enchilada sauce.
- Fill the tortilla with the meat mixture and fold it up.
- In a shallow pot, put the enchilada and, if desired, top with sauce and cheese.
- Bake till the cheese has dissolved and the enchiladas are golden brown, around 20 mins.

14. Chicken and Dumplings

Preparation time thirty-five mins Cooking Time eight hrs fifteen mins
Servings eight persons
Nutritional facts 401 calories Carb 32 gm Protein 45 gm Fat 10 gm Sodium 146 mg Potassium 940 mg Phosphorous 584 mg
Ingredients

- 2 cups of water or low salt chicken broth
- 1 whole chicken or 3 lbs. of sliced chicken
- 2 cups of flour
- 1/2 teaspoon of mace or nutmeg
- 3 teaspoons of baking powder
- 1/2 teaspoon of black pepper
- 1/4 cup of flour
- 2 eggs
- 2/3 cup of milk
- 1 stalk of celery with leaves, cut fine
- 2 tablespoons of unsalted margarine or butter
- 2-3 sliced carrots

Instructions

- Chicken, spices, vegetables and water or broth are to be put in slow cooker.
- More water just enough to cover chicken by around one inch should be included.
- Cooker should be flipped on low for around 6-8 hrs.
- It should be removed to an oven proof dish.
- Then bones can be removed, if desired.
- It should be covered and kept warm.
- Then slow cooker should be flipped to high flame. Include the quarter cup flour and stir quickly, to avoid lumps.
- Using knives cut the butter into the two cups of flour.
- Then it should be blended wet Ingredients to stiff dough. Now drop in spoonfuls into the boiling broth.
- The cooked should be covered while reducing the flame to prevent boiling. It should be cooked for 15 mins without removing the lid.
- Then chicken should be put in big-sized serving dish and thickened sauce is to be put. Serve with dumplings.

15. Chicken Lasagna with White Sauce

Preparation time fourteen mins Cooking Time fifty-eight mins
Servings six persons

Nutritional facts 453 calories Carb 32 gm Protein 23 gm Fat 5 gm Sodium 277 mg Potassium 317 mg Phosphorous 179 mg

Ingredients

- 1 1/2 cups of Mocha Mix (or any other non-dairy creamer)
- 1/4 cup of white wine (optional)
- 1 package of no boil lasagna noodles
- 6 ounces of chicken (thigh or breast)
- 1 tablespoon of oregano
- 1/4 teaspoon of black pepper
- 1/2 cup of mushrooms, thick sliced
- 12 ounces of low sodium chicken broth
- 3 tablespoons of flour
- 1/2 cup of grated fresh parmesan cheese
- 6 ounces of cream cheese
- 1/4 cup of olive oil
- 1 big diced onion
- 1/4~1/2 teaspoon of nutmeg
- 1 1/2 zucchini, sliced into tiny moons

Instructions

- Warm up your oven at 375 º F.
- Bring the chicken and stock to the boil in a small-sized pot and then flip to a low flame and continue to cook till the chicken is white as well as fully cooked. If you cut the chicken into pieces, it will cook faster.
- Meanwhile, warm olive oil, oregano, onion, and black pepper inside a big-sized sauté pot on moderate flame for 5 mins, or till onion begins to tendered.
- Whisk in the mushrooms.
- To disseminate flavors, evenly sprinkle flour over pot and stir. The Ingredients in the pot should clump simultaneously.
- Allow for another few mins (3 mins) of cooking time.
- Break up the cream cheese and stir it into the pot till it melts and is evenly distributed. (around 2 mins)
- Slowly put in the Mocha mix, stirring constantly.
- Ingredients should thicken but not clump simultaneously. Continue stirring if the mixture is still clumpy.
- Nutmeg should be included at this point.
- Stir in the parmesan cheese and continue to boil for another five min, till the sauce has thickened.
- Remove the chicken from the pot (reserve the broth) and shred it with two forks, trying to keep the pieces even.
- To thin out the cream mixture, include in 1/2 cup of rest of the broth, stirring occasionally for two min.
- Put lasagna sheets in pot, top with 1/3 of the sauce, 1/2 of the chicken, and half of the zucchini slices (equally distributed on top); repeat layers, finishing with the rest of the sauce.
- Cover using foil and bake for around 30 mins, removing foil for the last few mins till desired crispiness is achieved.

16. Chicken Seafood Gumbo

Preparation time nine mins Cooking Time thirty-seven mins
Servings twelve persons

Nutritional facts 240 calories Carb 19 gm Protein 10 gm Fat 2 gm Sodium 320 mg Potassium 426 mg Phosphorous 156 mg

Ingredients

- 8 ounces of lean smoked turkey sausage, sliced
- 1 tablespoon of canola oil
- 1 tablespoon of salt-free Cajun seasoning
- 1/2 pound of cooked shrimp
- 6 ounces of tinned crab, drained
- 1 sliced yellow onion
- 2 sliced skinless chicken breasts
- 1/2 cup of canola oil
- 2 quarts of low sodium chicken broth
- 1/2 cup of flour
- 3 sliced celery stalks
- 1 sliced red bell pepper
- 3 cups of frozen sliced okra

Instructions

- In a 4.5 quart or bigger pot, warm 1 tsp canola oil over moderate flame.
- Cook for 10 mins with bell pepper, celery, chicken, onion, as well as sausage.
- Take the mixture out of the pot and leave it aside.
- Diminish to a moderate flame setting.
- To create a roux, include half cup canola oil and mix in flour.
- Cook for another min or two after including the Cajun seasoning.
- Stir in the chicken broth carefully, continually stirring to avoid lumps.
- Raise the flame to moderate-high as well as bring the mixture to the boil, stirring occasionally, for around 10 mins, or till it thickens mildly.
- Diminish flame to moderate and mix in the crab, shrimp, and okra, as well as the chicken mixture.
- You need to cook for 10 mins, or till thoroughly heated.

17. Chinese Chicken Salad

Preparation time twelve mins Cooking Time eighteen mins
Servings eight persons
Nutritional facts 203 calories Carb 13 gm Protein 19 gm Fat 5 gm Sodium 48 mg Potassium 259 mg Phosphorous 41 mg

Ingredients

- 3 tablespoons of divided olive oil
- 2 packages of ramen noodles
- 1/4 cup of sugar or Splenda
- 2 cups of cooked chicken or turkey, diced
- 1 tablespoon of sesame oil
- 1/2 head of cabbage, shredded & sliced
- 4 green onions, diced
- 2 tablespoons of sesame seeds
- 1/2 cup of rice vinegar or white wine vinegar

Instructions

- Take the ramen noodles out of the packet and smash them.
- Remove the seasoning packets from the packages.

- In a griddle, warm 1 tbsp. oil.
- Mix the dried noodles as well as sesame seeds inside a mixing container.
- Toast till golden brown on both sides.
- Inside a container, mix the cabbage, chicken or turkey, and green onions, then include the ramen noodles and sesame seeds.
- Inside a separate container, mix the sesame oil, sugar, 2 tsps. of oil, and vinegar.
- Drizzle the dressing over the salad.

18. Confetti Chicken 'N Rice

Preparation time fourteen mins Cooking Time thirty-five mins
Servings four persons
Nutritional facts 519 calories Carb 80 gm Protein 17 gm Fat 6 gm Sodium 37 mg Potassium 316 mg Phosphorous 152 mg
Ingredients
- 1 tablespoon of cumin
- 3 tablespoons of olive oil, divided
- 1/2 teaspoon of black pepper
- 1 fresh cubed zucchini
- 1/4 teaspoon of cayenne pepper
- 1 big red bell pepper, cubed
- 2 teaspoons Mrs. of the Dash original
- 1 moderate diced red onion
- 1/2 teaspoon of garlic powder
- 1 boneless & skinless chicken breast
- 3 ears, kernels removed or around 2 1/4 cups of no salt included frozen corn
- 1 package of Uncle Ben's original ready rice

Instructions
- Two tablespoons olive oil is heated in a big-sized nonstick griddle over moderate high flame.
- Carefully slide the chicken breast into the griddle while the oil is heated.
- Remove the chicken from the pot when the juices have run clean (around 15 mins).
- Then one tablespoon olive oil, zucchini, red pepper, maize, and onion are included in the same griddle
- Sauté the onions on moderate to moderate high flame till they begin to caramelize (around 10 mins).
- Include garlic powder, black pepper, cumin, Mrs. Dash, as well as cayenne pepper after that.
- Reflip the cubed chicken to the pot with the veggies, lower flame to moderate low, and stir for around 5 mins.
- Follow the rice package's Instructions.
- When the rice is done, mix it with the veggies and cook for some more mins.

19. Cowboy Caviar Bean and Rice Salad

Preparation time fifteen mins Cooking Time one hr twelve mins
Servings six persons
Nutritional facts 237 calories Carb 34 gm Protein 4 gm Fat 5 gm Sodium 101 mg Potassium 195 mg Phosphorous 40 mg
Ingredients
- 1/2 cup of olive or canola oil
- 1/2 cup of fresh or frozen corn, cooked
- 1 jalapeño, seeded and diced

- 1/2 cup of red bell pepper, diced
- 1/2 cup of low salt tinned black beans, drained & washed
- 2 tablespoons of brown sugar
- 1 tablespoon of Dijon mustard
- 1/2 teaspoon of black pepper
- 3 cups of cooked rice
- 1/4 cup of lime juice
- 1/2 cup of sliced cilantro

Instructions
- Rice and corn are to be prepared first. Then let cool.
- Whisk brown sugar, mustard, lime juice, oil, and black pepper simultaneously for making the dressing.
- All other Ingredients are to be mixed inside a big-sized container.
- Dressing is to be put over salad and stirred.
- It should be chilled for one hr in fridge.

20. Creamy Tuna Twist

Preparation time thirty mins Cooking Time zero mins
Servings four persons
Nutritional facts 421 calories Carb 20 gm Protein 15 gm Fat 31 gm Sodium 379 mg Potassium 204 mg Phosphorous 122 mg
Ingredients
- Half cup of cooked peas
- One and a half cups of cooked shell macaroni
- 3/4 cup of mayonnaise
- 1 can (6 1/2 ounces) of tuna, water packed and drained
- Two tablespoons of vinegar
- 1/2 cup of celery, sliced into pea size
- One tbsp. of dried dill weed

Instructions
- Stir vinegar, Mayonnaise, and macaroni shells are to be stirred inside a big-sized container till smooth.
- Then rest of the components are included and stirred till mixed.
- Cover and let chill.

21. Crock Pot Chili Verde

Preparation time fourteen mins Cooking Time seven hrs thirty mins
Servings six to eight persons
Nutritional facts 227 calories Carb 36 gm Protein 6 gm Fat 10 gm Sodium 43 mg Potassium 222 mg Phosphorous 83 mg
Ingredients
- 3/4 teaspoon of garlic powder
- one jar (sixteen oz.) of Green Tomatillo Salsa or two cups of fresh tomatillos plus half cup of vinegar
- half cup of low-sodium beef broth
- one green bell pepper sliced into one-inch squares
- one and a half tablespoons of corn starch
- 2 big onions, wedges
- 1/2-3/4 teaspoon of red chili flakes
- two and two and a half pounds of pork or pork loin slices, trim the fat

- 1 red bell pepper cut into one-inch squares

Instructions

- Pork slices, tomatillos or green tomatillo sauce, & onions are to be layered in a 4-quart slow cooker.
- Cornstarch is mixed into broth and then included to crock pot with garlic powder, vinegar and red chili flakes.
- It should be covered and cooked on low for six and a half- seven hrs or till the pork is soft.
- The flame setting is to be increased to high.
- Green and red bell peppers are stirred in.
- It should be covered and cooked on high for 15 min to 1/2 hr.
- Can be served with rice, or put across low salt corn chips.

22. Crock Pot White Chicken Chili

Preparation time fourteen mins Cooking Time eleven hrs ten mins
Servings twelve to fourteen persons
Nutritional facts 306 calories Carb 32 gm Protein 25 gm Fat 12 gm Sodium 75 mg Potassium 845 mg Phosphorous 321 mg

Ingredients

- 1 cup of dried black-eyed peas
- 1 cup of dried Great Northern beans
- 2 teaspoons of oregano
- 1 teaspoon of black pepper
- 8 cups of water
- 2 moderate diced onions
- three tbsps. of crushed garlic
- two lbs. of chicken breast, chopped
- one to two jalapeño chili peppers, chopped
- two tbsps. of vegetable oil or canola
- 1 cup of dried lima beans
- 2 teaspoons of cumin
- half cup of dried small lima beans
- 2 cups of frozen corn
- half tsp. of cayenne pepper
- two cups of sour cream

Instructions

- The dried beans are to be washed and sorted.
- Beans are to be put in Crock-Pot (slow cooker) with water.
- Temp. should be set at low.
- Sauté diced chicken, onions, garlic, and jalapeños in vegetable or canola oil in a griddle for 10 mins, till mildly browned.
- Include to the Crock-Pot.
- Corn and spices are included to mixture.
- Allow it to cook for around 9-11 hrs, or overnight.
- Prior to serving, sour cream can be stirred in.

23. Curry Chicken Salad

Preparation time twelve mins Cooking Time zero mins
Servings eight persons
Nutritional facts 304 calories Carb 25 gm Protein 21 gm Fat 10 gm Sodium 231 mg Potassium 361 mg Phosphorous 65 mg

Ingredients

- 1 teaspoon of curry powder
- 1 1/2 cups or 3/4 cup of every mayonnaise or light sour cream
- 3 celery stalks, sliced
- 2 cups of cooked chicken or turkey
- 1/2 cup of raisins
- 4 sliced green onions
- 1/2 cup of nuts (sliced almonds, cashews, hazelnuts, or pecans)
- 1/2 cup of low sodium Mango Chutney

Instructions

- Mayo, curry powder, and chutney are blended to create dressing.
- Inside a container whisk Chicken, nuts, celery, green onions, and raisins are whisked inside a container. Then the dressing is mixed into this mixture.
- Let it chill overnight in the fridge for more flavor.

24. Dijon Chicken

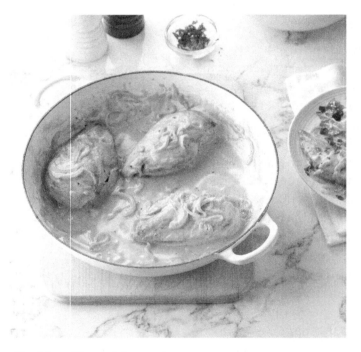

Preparation time five mins Cooking Time thirty mins
Servings four persons
Nutritional facts 189 calories Carb 14 gm Protein 25 gm Fat 14 gm Sodium 258 mg Potassium 454 mg Phosphorous 250 mg
Ingredients

- One teaspoon of lemon Juice
- Four boneless chicken breasts
- 3 tablespoons of honey
- Quarter cup of Dijon mustard
- 1 teaspoon of curry powder

Instructions

- Heat oven at 350 º F.
- Put chicken in a baking dish.
- Mix other components inside a container.
- Both sides of chicken are to be brushed with sauce.

- It should be baked for 30 mins or till a chicken's internal temperature is 165 º F.

25. Dilled Fish

Preparation time five mins Cooking Time twenty mins
Servings six persons
Nutritional facts 112 calories Carb 1 gm Protein 23 gm Fat 5 gm Sodium 63 mg Potassium 350 mg
Phosphorous 194 mg
Ingredients

- 1 1/2 pounds of fresh, firm white fish
- A dash of pepper
- One teaspoon of instant (freeze dried) onion, minced
- 1/2 teaspoon of dill weed
- Four teaspoons of lemon juice
- Quarter teaspoon of mustard powder

Instructions

- Heat oven at 475 º F.
- Fish should be washed and dried.
- Put in baking dish.
- Mix onion, dill weed, mustard, and pepper in 2 tbsps. of water.
- Lemon juice is included to spice and put evenly over fish.
- It should be baked uncovered for 17-20 mins.

26. Fast Fajitas

Preparation time twelve hrs Cooking Time twenty mins
Servings four persons
Nutritional facts 320 calories Carb 34 gm Protein 29 gm Fat 5 gm Sodium 142 mg Potassium 445 mg
Phosphorous 332 mg
Ingredients

- 1 lemon juice & zest of lemon or orange
- sour cream as required
- 1 tablespoon of olive oil
- 8 corn tortillas
- dash of cayenne pepper
- 1 pound of meat, tofu, shrimp, bite size pieces
- 1 lime juice & zest of lime
- 1 sliced onion
- 2 sliced bell peppers
- 1 teaspoon of cumin
- cilantro as required

Instructions

- Oil, citrus zest and juice, cayenne pepper and cumin are to be included inside a small-sized container to create the marinade.
- Vegetables, meat, and marinade are to be put in a bag or shallow dish and marinated overnight.
- Then marinated meat and vegetables are to be cooked in a big-sized griddle at moderate flame till the onions become tender and begin to caramelize (flip light brown) as well as the meat is cooked through. This should take 15-20 mins.
- It should be served in tortillas and topped with sour cream and cilantro.

27. Fast Roast Chicken with Lemon & Herbs

Preparation time nine mins Cooking Time thirty-five mins
Servings four persons
Nutritional facts 231 calories Carb 0 gm Protein 19 gm Fat 0 gm Sodium 77 mg Potassium 222 mg
Phosphorous 188 mg
Ingredients

- 2 cloves of peeled and crushed garlic
- One (4-5 pounds) of whole chicken, fresh or thawed
- Two and a half tablespoons of sliced fresh herbs (thyme, sage, etc.)
- One small finely sliced lemon
- Two tablespoons of tendered and unsalted butter
- 1 tablespoon of olive oil

Instructions

- Heat oven at 450 ° F.
- Put the chicken in a roasting pot.
- Herbs, butter and garlic are to be mixed simultaneously inside a small-sized container.
- Put the herbed butter inside the body cavity of the chicken, along with the lemon slices.
- The olive oil is to be rubbed over the skin of the bird.
- Should be roasted for 15 mins per pound, or till internal temperature reaches 165 ° F.
- The buttery juices and slices of lemon are to be drained and put over chicken.
- Allow the chicken to rest for 20 mins prior to carving.

28. Fresh Marinara Sauce

Preparation time fourteen mins Cooking Time twelve mins
Servings sixteen persons
Nutritional facts 80 calories Carb 9 gm Protein 2 gm Fat 3 gm Sodium 25 mg Potassium 341 mg
Phosphorous 46 mg
Ingredients

- 1 pot of boiling water
- six lbs. or fifteen moderate ripe tomatoes or two to twenty-eight oz. cans low salt tomatoes
- one tablespoon of dry or 3 tablespoons of fresh oregano
- 2 big sliced onions
- one-third cup olive oil
- two tbsps. of dry or one-third cup of fresh basil, sliced
- 3-4 big grated carrots
- 6 garlic cloves, minced
- 1 teaspoon of pepper

Instructions

- Place in boiling water fresh tomatoes a few at a time, and conceal for around one min.
- These should be lifted out with slotted spatula and plunged into cold water.
- Skins should be peeled off and tomatoes to be coarsely sliced to get eleven-twelve cups.
- Tinned low sodium tomatoes should be coarsely sliced.
- Onion, garlic, and carrots are cooked in a five-quart kettle in oil across moderate flame, mixing irregularly, till onions are translucent.
- Then tomatoes, oregano, basil, and pepper are included.
- Raise to the boil.
- Then lower the flame and simmer frequently, uncovered, mixing irregularly till sauce denses. It should be served over pasta.
- Extra sauce should be frozen in freezer bowls or food storage bags till required.

29. Fruit Vinegar Chicken

Preparation time eight mins Cooking Time fifty mins
Servings six persons
Nutritional facts 413 calories Carb 3 gm Protein 28 gm Fat 3 gm Sodium 106 mg Potassium 335 mg
Phosphorous 227 mg
Ingredients

- Half a teaspoon of basil
- 2 pounds of chicken
- Half cup of fruit or berry vinegar
- Quarter cup of orange juice
- Half a teaspoon of marjoram
- 1/4 cup of oil
- Half a teaspoon of tarragon

Instructions

- Heat oven at 350 º F.
- Then all Ingredients are to be mixed in a big-sized zip lock bag.
- It should be marinade for 15-20 mins in the fridge.
- Chicken should be removed from bag, and put in a baking dish.
- It should be baked for thirty mins or till a chicken's internal temperature is 165 º F.

30. Fruity Chicken Salad

Preparation time nine mins Cooking Time zero mins
Servings eight persons
Nutritional facts 279 calories Carb 20 gm Protein 15 gm Fat 2 gm Sodium 82 mg Potassium 352 mg
Phosphorous 159 mg
Ingredients

- 1 sliced green onion
- 2 cups of chicken breasts, cooked and cubed
- 1 teaspoon of rice vinegar, unseasoned
- 1 apple, cubed
- 3/4 cup of raisins
- 1/2 cup of sour cream
- 2 teaspoons of sugar
- 1/4 cup of mayo
- 1 cup of sliced almonds
- 2 cups of seedless grapes
- 1 sliced stalk celery
- 1/2 teaspoon of Chinese Five-Spice Blend

Instructions

- Chicken, apples, celery, green onion, almonds, grapes, and raisins are to be mixed inside a big-sized container.
- Sour cream, sugar, rice vinegar, mayo, and Chinese Five-Spice Blend are to be mixed inside a separate container.
- Dressing is mixed into chicken mixture.

31. Grilled Lemon Chicken Kebabs

Preparation time twelve hrs Cooking Time ten mins
Servings two persons
Nutritional facts 362 calories Carb 6 gm Protein 27 gm Fat 0 gm Sodium 119 mg Potassium 404 mg
Phosphorous 238 mg

Ingredients

- 3 tablespoons of olive oil
- 4 pieces of boneless and skinless chicken thighs
- 1 peeled and crushed clove of garlic
- 2 bay leaves, torn in 1/2
- 1 tablespoon of sliced fresh herbs (thyme, sage, etc.)
- 2 lemons
- 1 teaspoon of white wine vinegar

Instructions

- Every thigh is to be sliced into chunky pieces and put inside a container.
- One tsp lemon zest and juice are to be grated in the rest of the whole lemon.
- It should be included to the chicken along with the oil, garlic, herbs and vinegar.
- It should be covered and marinated for around three hrs, or for overnight.
- The other lemon is to be sliced into 4 thick slices and then every slice is to be cut into 4 pieces.
- The lemon slices and the chicken pieces are to be alternated on a wooden skewer. Repeat for every skewer, packing them as tightly as possible, and finishing with a lemon slice.
- It should be grilled in the oven, barbecue, or countertop grill till done, roughly ten mins per side.

32. Grilled Salmon with Fruit Salsa

Preparation time five mins Cooking Time eight mins
Servings four persons
Nutritional facts 374 calories Carb 3 gm Protein 38 gm Fat 2 gm Sodium 110 mg Potassium 287 mg Phosphorous 219 mg

Ingredients

- 2 tablespoons of black pepper
- 4 (6 ounces every) of salmon fillets, skin on
- 1 tablespoon of dried thyme
- 2 1/2 teaspoons of paprika
- 4 tablespoons of olive oil, divided
- 2 tablespoons of garlic powder
- 1 tablespoon of onion powder
- 2 teaspoons of creole seasoning
- 1 tablespoon of cayenne pepper
- 1/2 teaspoon of black pepper
- 1 tablespoon of dried oregano
- Fruit Salsa as required

Instructions

- Both sides of the salmon are to be brushed with olive oil and seasoned with creole seasoning & pepper.
- Put fish on the grill skin side down. Then cook for three mins. Next, flip fish 45 º and cook for another three mins.
- Fish is to be flipped again and cooked for 2 mins or till cooked through to desired doneness.
- Fish should be removed from grill and served with fruit salsa spooned over the fish.
- Should be served immediately.

33. Grilled Vegetable Pasta Salad

Preparation time nine mins Cooking Time fifteen mins
Servings eight persons
Nutritional facts 242 calories Carb 37 gm Protein 7 gm Fat 14 gm Sodium 76 mg Potassium 294 mg Phosphorous 102mg

Ingredients

- 1 tablespoon & 1 teaspoon of Dijon mustard
- 2 minced garlic cloves
- 1 moderate sliced red onion
- 12 ounces of rotini, uncooked
- 2 moderate sliced zucchini
- 1/4 cup of lemon juice
- 2 tablespoons of fresh basil leaves, shredded
- 1 head of anise (fennel), sliced
- 8 quartered mushrooms
- 1/4 cup of olive oil
- 1 tablespoon of fresh thyme
- One tablespoon of sliced fresh parsley
- 1/2 teaspoon of black pepper

Instructions

- The dressing (garlic through black pepper) is made by including all of the Ingredients simultaneously inside a mixing container and whisking them simultaneously.
- All the vegetables are to be included inside a big-sized mixing container. Then half of dressing is to be put over the vegetables and stirred till all are mildly coated. Allow the vegetables to marinate while the pasta is being cooked following package directions. Pasta should be washed in cold water.
- Switch the oven on to broil. Use a greased broiler pot if using the oven.
- Then the vegetables are to be spread on broiling pot & cook till the vegetables flip golden brown. Should be stirred every 4-5 mins to allow the browning to occur evenly. When browned, it should be put into a big-sized serving container. Pasta should be included and the rest of the dressing, and fresh herbs.

34. Herb Breaded Chicken

Preparation time five mins Cooking Time twenty-fifty mins
Servings four persons
Nutritional facts 172 calories Carb 7 gm Protein 27 gm Fat 10 gm Sodium 180 mg Potassium 444 mg Phosphorous 249 mg
Ingredients

- 1 1/2 slices of whole wheat bread
- 1/4 teaspoon of basil
- Quarter teaspoon of thyme
- 1/4 teaspoon of oregano
- Quarter teaspoon of tarragon
- Quarter teaspoon of ground black pepper
- 1/4 teaspoon of paprika
- One pound of boneless chicken breasts

Instructions

- Heat oven at 400 º F.
- Mix Herbs and spices are to be mixed inside mixer or food processor with bread.
- It should be mixed well.
- Chicken is to be dipped in an herb mixture.
- It should be baked in a single layer for 20 mins (boneless chicken) or 50 mins (bone-in).

35. Honey Herb Glazed Turkey

Preparation time thirty mins Cooking Time twenty-five mins
Servings six persons
Nutritional facts 412 calories Carb 7 gm Protein 49 gm Fat 18 gm Sodium 119 mg Potassium 526 mg
Phosphorous 357 mg
Ingredients

- 2 celery stalks, whole
- 10-12 pounds of whole turkey
- 2 teaspoons of celery seed
- 1/2 cup of unsalted butter
- one-third cup of fresh thyme stripped from the stems (around fourteen stems)
- two tablespoons of fresh sage leaves
- one onion, sliced into wedges
- two fresh bay leaves
- one lemon, sliced into chunks
- quarter cup of honey
- one-third cup of olive oil
- two teaspoons of lemon juice

Instructions

- Warm up your oven at 350 º F.
- Neck and giblets are to be removed from turkey.
- Turkey should be filled using onion, celery and lemon.
- Skin should be rubbed with olive oil.
- Place on two sheets of aluminum foil.
- The top of bird should be covered with separate sheet of foil, which can be removed later.
- The edges of the foil are to be sealed and put on a rack and roasted in the oven.
- During the process of turkey cooking, slice thyme and sage leaves finely.
- Next sliced herbs, bay leaves, and honey are included to butter.
- It should be simmered for 10 mins, till butter is mildly browned. Then the bay leaves should be removed.
- The oven temperature should be raised to 500 º F when the turkey attains temperature of 145-155 º F. The top foil should be removed. Then baste turkey with honey herb mixture, every five to ten mins or so.
- When the turkey attains a temperature of 160 º F, it should be removed from oven. Then tent with foil and allow it to rest for thirty mins prior to carving.

36. Low Salt Stir-Fry

Preparation time nine mins Cooking Time twelve mins
Servings two persons
Nutritional facts 231 calories Carb 13 gm Protein 14 gm Fat 28 gm Sodium 355 mg Potassium 442 mg
Phosphorous 54 mg
Ingredients

- 1/2 cup of white wine vinegar or rice vinegar
- Four cups (around 3/4 pound) of mixed greens (collard, lettuce, beet, etc.)
- 8 ounces of tofu, cut into cubes
- 1 cup of onions, sliced thin
- Half teaspoon of sesame oil
- 1 tablespoon of low sodium soy sauce
- 1/4 teaspoon of curry powder
- 1 tablespoon of olive oil
- 1/2 teaspoon of sesame seeds

Instructions
- Greens should be cut into two-inch-long shreds.
- Warm up oil in a sauté pot.
- Sauté onions till translucent, for 2 mins.
- Curry should be sprinkled over onions and sugar and greens are to be included.
- It should be covered.
- Flame should be diminished and allow greens to steam in their own juice till tender, for 5-8 mins. Never overcook as greens will flip darker.
- The greens should be removed with slotted spoon leaving juices in pot.
- Soy sauce and vinegar are included and heated to boiling.
- When sauce is mildly thickened, it should be removed from flame and put over greens.
- It should be garnished with sesame oil and seeds.

37. Mac in a Flash (Macaroni & Cheese)

Preparation time five mins Cooking Time eight mins
Servings four persons
Nutritional facts 152 calories Carb18 gm Protein 7 gm Fat 35 gm Sodium 90 mg Potassium 52 mg Phosphorous 107 mg
Ingredients
- One teaspoon of unsalted butter
- 1 cup of uncooked noodles, any shape
- 1/2 cup of grated cheddar cheese
- Three cups of water
- Quarter teaspoon of dry ground mustard
Instructions
- Water should be boiled. Noodles should be included and cooked for 5-7 mins or till tender.
- Noodles should be drained.
- Then sprinkle noodles with cheese.
- Next, stir in butter and ground mustard.

38. Marinated Shrimp & Pasta Salad

Preparation time five hrs Cooking Time twenty-five mins
Servings ten persons
Nutritional facts 473 calories Carb 65 gm Protein 16 gm Fat 4 gm Sodium 143 mg Potassium 312 mg Phosphorous 117 mg
Ingredients
- 1/2 big diced red bell pepper
- 12 ounces of uncooked tri-color pasta
- one tbsp. of Dijon mustard
- half tsp. of garlic powder
- 15-20 baby carrots, cut into thick rounds
- 1/2 teaspoon of black pepper
- one and a half cups of cauliflower, dime size pieces
- half pound of cooked shrimp
- 1/4 cup of honey
- 1/2 English cucumber, cubed
- 1/4 cup of balsamic vinegar
- 1/2 big diced yellow bell pepper
- 4 diced stalks celery
- 3/4 cup of olive oil

- 1/2 diced red onion

Instructions

- Pasta is to be cooked according to package Instructions. It should be washed and drained under cold water to cool quickly.
- During the cooking process, cut up vegetables as well as put into a big-sized mixing container. Then include the shrimp.
- Honey, mustard, black pepper, vinegar, and garlic powder are to be whisked inside a small-sized mixing container.
- During the whisking, gradually include the oil and whisk everything simultaneously.
- Then cooled pasta is included to the container with the vegetables and shrimp. Then mix them all gently.
- The marinade is to be put over the pasta mixture and gently whisked for an even coat.
- It should be covered with plastic wrap and refrigerated around 5 hrs.
- It should be stirred and served chilled.

39. Mashed Cauliflower Potatoes

Preparation time twelve mins Cooking Time fourteen mins
Servings four persons
Nutritional facts 83 calories Carb 7 gm Protein 2 gm Fat 4 gm Sodium 67 mg Potassium 282 mg Phosphorous 52 mg
Ingredients

- Two tablespoons of margarine
- One moderate red potato
- Quarter cup of sliced onion
- 8 ounces of cauliflower florets
- One teaspoon of dried parsley
- 1/4 teaspoon of garlic powder
- pepper as required

Instructions

- Potato, parsley, onion, cauliflower, and garlic powder are to be mixed inside a moderate-sized saucepot with sufficient water to cover.
- It should be brought to the boil on high and then flame is to be diminished to simmer.
- It should be cooked for 12 mins or till vegetables are tender.
- It should be drained well.
- It should be mashed using potato masher.
- Margarine should be included and mashed till smooth.
- Then include pepper as required.

40. Mashed Parsnips

Preparation time nine mins Cooking Time thirty-nine mins
Servings six persons
Nutritional facts 252 calories Carb 37 gm Protein 4 gm Fat 21 gm Sodium 129 mg Potassium 831 mg Phosphorous 135 mg
Ingredients

- Half cup of sour cream, half and half or yogurt
- 3-4 big parsnips
- 1/2 cup of butter
- Three to four big potatoes (russets are best)
- Five to seven fresh sage leaves

Instructions

- Parsnips should be peeled. If they're really big, cut out the woody core; if they're small, they'll be fine.
- Microwave for 10-12 mins, or till done, in a microwave-safe dish.
- Meanwhile, cut the potatoes in half and boil them in a pot till they are fork tender, around 10-15 mins.
- Drain thoroughly.
- For one to two mins in butter, sauté sage leaves.
- Inside a mixing container, mix the parsnips and potatoes, whip using an electric mixer or mash using a potato masher, and stir in the sage butter and sour cream or half-and-half.
- Blend till completely smooth.

41. Master Ground Beef Mix

Preparation time twelve mins Cooking Time twenty-four mins
Servings eight persons
Nutritional facts 331 calories Carb 13 gm Protein 32 gm Fat 4 gm Sodium 215 mg Potassium 482 mg Phosphorous 256 mg
Ingredients
- 1 teaspoon of garlic powder
- 2 pounds of ground beef
- 1/4 teaspoon of pepper
- 1 teaspoon of Italian seasoning
- 1/2 cup of milk
- 4 slices of white bread, cubed
- 1 cup of diced onion
- 3 tablespoons of Worcestershire sauce

Instructions
- Mix simultaneously all Ingredients in a big-sized fry pot on the stove top.
- Cook till the meat is no longer red, stirring occasionally.
- Remove the meat from the flame and drain any rest of the liquid.
- Allow to cool in the fridge.
- One cup of meat is to be portioned into freezer containers or freezer weight bags.
- For later use it should be frozen for tacos, Shepherd's pie, stroganoff, nachos, soups, goulash and casseroles later.
- In the freezer, it lasts 3 months.

42. Mediterranean Lamb Patties

Preparation time three mins Cooking Time twelve mins
Servings four persons
Nutritional facts 305 calories Carb 5 gm Protein 19 gm Fat 12 gm Sodium 229 mg Potassium 40 mg Phosphorous 145 mg
Ingredients
- 1/2 cup of crumbled feta cheese
- 1 lb. of ground lamb
- 1/2 teaspoon of ground pepper
- 1 teaspoon of dried oregano (or dried mint)
- 1/4 cup of onion, finely sliced
- 1 clove of garlic, finely sliced
- 1/4 cup of panko bread crumbs
- 1 whole egg

Instructions

- Mix simultaneously all of the Ingredients inside a big-sized mixing container and stir well.
- Form into four 1/2-inch thick patties of equal size.
- Over moderate-high flame, warm up a big-sized nonstick griddle.
- Include patties and cook on high flame till browned, around 5 mins per side, prior to flipping and flipping off the flame.
- Create sure the patties are fully cooked, the internal temperature has risen to 160 º F, and it is no longer pink in the middle.

43. Mediterranean Pizza

Preparation time five mins Cooking Time fifteen mins
Servings twelve persons
Nutritional facts 176 calories Carb 18 gm Protein 7 gm Fat 0 gm Sodium 240 mg Potassium 86 mg Phosphorous 90 mg
Ingredients

- Two garlic cloves, sliced finely
- 1 crust, 2 pitas readymade pizza dough or big pitas
- One sliced roma tomato
- Ten finely sliced basil leaves
- One tablespoon of olive oil
- 3 ounces of goat cheese, or ricotta

Instructions

- Warm up your oven at 450 º F.
- Apply olive oil to the pizza crust.
- Garlic slices should be evenly distributed across the crust.
- Tomato slices should be used to cover the garlic cloves.
- Basil should be evenly distributed across the pizza, followed by goat cheese.
- Bake for 10-15 mins in the oven, or according to the crust package Instructions.

44. Mediterranean Roasted Red Pepper Soup

Preparation time nine mins Cooking Time thirty-two mins
Servings six persons
Nutritional facts 240 calories Carb 31 gm Protein 11 gm Fat 5 gm Sodium 128 mg Potassium 370 mg Phosphorous 83 mg
Ingredients

- 6 garlic of cloves, minced
- 2 tablespoons of olive oil
- 1 tablespoon of red wine vinegar
- 1/2 cup of lentils, washed & sorted
- 3 fresh roasted red peppers
- 1 teaspoon of paprika
- 1 (28 ounces) can of diced tomatoes
- 2 cups of low salt chicken broth or water
- 2/3 cup of nonfat dry milk
- 2 big onions, diced
- 1/4 cup of almonds or cashews, toasted

Instructions

- Warm the olive oil, then include the onions and cook, stirring occasionally, till they are tender and caramelized.

- Cook for 2 mins after including the garlic and paprika.
- One cup broth, peppers, lentils, and tomatoes are to be included next.
- Bring to boil, then flip to a low flame and cover to keep the lentils warm till they are tender (around 30 min).
- Blend or process the soup in batches till it is completely smooth.
- To the last batch, include vinegar and dry milk.
- Mix simultaneously all Ingredients inside a mixing container.
- If the soup needs more flavor, then you need to season using more vinegar and if it's too thick, put a small amount of broth.
- If desired, garnish with a sprinkling of cashews or almonds and a drizzle of oil.

45. New England Clam-Chowder

Preparation time two hrs thirteen mins Cooking Time thirty mins
Servings six persons
Nutritional facts 232 calories Carb 24 gm Protein 14 gm Fat 5 gm Sodium 111 mg Potassium 749 mg Phosphorous 272 mg
Ingredients
- quarter cup margarine
- half cup sliced onion
- three tablespoons flour
- half cup sliced celery
- quarter teaspoon pepper
- one (6-1/2) ounce can of sliced clams
- two cups of raw potatoes, sliced in half-inch cubes
- paprika for the garnish
- 3 cups of milk

Instructions
- Soak cubed potatoes for 2 hrs in four cups cold water.
- Drain and include it to the soup as directed.
- In a 2-quart saucepot, melt margarine and sauté celery and onion till tender.
- Sliced clams with juice, diced potatoes, and approximately three cups of milk are included to the pot.
- Cook for 5-10 mins.
- Mix 1/4 cup flour and milk inside a mixing container; stir into the hot chowder mixture.
- Include the pepper and continue to cook for another 15-20 mins to blend the flavors.
- Stir the mixture frequently.
- Paprika should be sprinkled over every serving.

46. Orange-Glazed Chicken

Preparation time fourteen mins Cooking Time thirty-seven mins
Servings six persons
Nutritional facts 262 calories Carb 15 gm Protein 24 gm Fat 5 gm Sodium 56 mg Potassium 353 mg Phosphorous 182 mg
Ingredients
- 6 chicken breast halves
- 1/4 cup oil
- quarter cup raisins

- one and a half cups orange Juice
- one-eighth tsp. nutmeg
- 1 dash ginger
- two tbsps. flour
- quarter tsp. cinnamon
- half cup mandarin orange (optional)

Instructions

- In a big-sized nonstick fry pot, warm the oil.
- Both sides of the chicken should be browned.
- Take out and reserve the chicken from the pot.
- Mix flour, ginger, nutmeg, and cinnamon inside a mixing container; include to hot oil.
- To create a smooth paste, whisk everything simultaneously quickly.
- Gradually put in the orange juice into the pot.
- Constantly stir.
- Cook for 3 mins at moderate flame till tender and thickened.
- Put the chicken back in the pot.
- Cook for 30 mins on low flame, or till chicken is tender as well as fully cooked.
- Include water to the sauce to thin it out if it is too thick.
- You need to heat till warm after including the mandarin orange slice.

47. Oven Blasted Vegetables

Preparation time twelve mins Cooking Time forty-nine mins
Servings six persons
Nutritional facts 247 calories Carb 40 gm Protein 5 gm Fat 5 gm Sodium 62 mg Potassium 243 mg Phosphorous 67 mg
Ingredients

- 3/4 cup of carrots
- 1 yukon gold potato
- 1 yam
- quarter cup fruit vinegar
- one beet
- two tbsps olive oil
- one onion
- as required parmesan cheese

Instructions

- Coin-shaped or lengthwise, cut vegetables into equal-sized pieces.
- You need to heat oil in a flat metal pot for two min in a 500°F oven.
- Cook for 10 mins after including the cubed potatoes, carrots, and onion.
- Cook for another 5 mins and then include the yam & beets and cook for another twenty mins, stirring every 10 mins.
- Remove from flame, season using parmesan cheese and vinegar, and serve.

48. Oven Fried Chicken

Preparation time thirty-six mins Cooking Time sixty mins
Servings eight persons
Nutritional facts 376 calories Carb 15 gm Protein 24 gm Fat 10 gm Sodium 109 mg Potassium 234 mg Phosphorous 172 mg
Ingredients

- half cup cornmeal
- quarter cup butter
- one tablespoon dried marjoram
- one tbsp. paprika
- one teaspoon ground mustard
- quarter cup corn oil
- one tablespoon dried tarragon
- half cup flour
- 4 pounds of whole chicken, sliced into parts
- one tsp. of ground pepper

Instructions

- Warm up your oven at 425 º F.
- In a 9 by 13-inch pot's lower part, melt quarter cup butter and quarter cup oil.
- Melt the butter and oil in the pot in the oven.
- In a big-sized zip lock plastic bag, mix half cup flour and half cup cornmeal while the butter and oil mixture is melting.
- You should season using salt & pepper.
- Shake in the chicken pieces.
- Put the pieces of chicken inside the hot oil, skin side down.
- It should be baked for thirty mins in the oven
- Turnover and bake for another 20-30 mins.

49. Louisiana BBQ Shrimp

Preparation time twelve mins Cooking Time thirty mins
Servings fifteen persons
Nutritional facts 420 calories Carb 6 gm Protein 35 gm Fat 5 gm Sodium 266 mg Potassium 223 mg Phosphorous 244 mg
Ingredients

- 1/4 cup of Worcestershire sauce
- 7.5 pounds of shrimp
- 2 teaspoons of oregano
- Two finely sliced lemons
- four garlic cloves, crushed
- quarter cup of lemon juice
- 2 tsps. of rosemary
- one tablespoon of parsley minced
- 2 teaspoons of paprika
- one cup olive oil
- half cup chili sauce
- two sticks butter
- Three teaspoons of cayenne pepper
- 1 teaspoon of Tabasco sauce

Instructions

- Shrimp should be peeled, deveined, and washed.
- Inside a sauce pan, mix the remaining components.
- Simmer for thirty mins on a low flame setting.
- In a small amount of olive oil, mildly sauté the shrimp till they are half cooked.
- Bring the BBQ sauce to a light boil over the shrimp.

- Serve with plenty of French bread inside a bread container or a regular container.

50. Rice Pudding with Cranberry Sauce

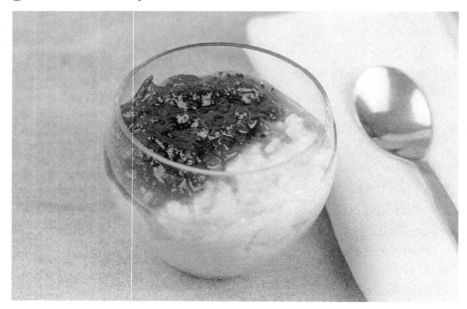

Preparation time nine mins Cooking Time thirty-nine mins
Servings six persons
Nutritional facts 184 calories Carb 32 gm Protein 5 gm Fat 4 gm Sodium 113 mg Potassium 125 mg Phosphorous 170 mg
Ingredients

- Half cup of whole berry cranberry sauce
- 3 cups of unsweetened almond milk
- Quarter cup of sugar
- 2 big eggs
- One cup of instant white rice
- 6 whole raw almonds
- One tsp. of vanilla extract
- Half a teaspoon of cinnamon

Instructions

- Mix rice, almond milk, and sugar inside a moderate-sized saucepot. On moderate-high flame, bring the combination to the boil. Constantly stir. Diminish to a low flame and cook for 6 mins. Remove the pot from the flame.
- Whisk simultaneously the eggs & vanilla extract inside a small-sized container. To temper the eggs and prevent them from curdling, whisk in a small amount of the hot almond milk as well as rice mixture.
- Stir constantly as you slowly put the egg mixture into the hot almond milk mixture.
- Reflip the saucepot to a low flame setting. You need to cook, stirring constantly, till the sauce has thickened, approximately 60 secs. Boiling is not recommended.
- Remove the pot from the flame & set it aside to cool for 30 mins.
- You need to put 1 almond inside the lower part of every container to serve. Fill 6 single-serving containers with rice pudding.
- Distribute the cranberry sauce among the six containers. Cinnamon should be sprinkled on top of the pudding.

51. Honey Apple Rice Cakes

Preparation time five mins Cooking Time zero mins
Servings two persons
Nutritional facts 140 calories Carb 24 gm Protein 2 gm Fat 4 gm Sodium 62 mg Potassium 147 mg
Phosphorous 55 mg
Ingredients

- 2 rice cakes
- One teaspoon of honey
- Two tbsps. of whipped cream cheese
- One moderate apple
- Two tsps. of pomegranate arils (optional)

Instructions

- Apple should be sliced into 10 wedges.
- One tablespoon of cream cheese should be spread on every rice cake.
- The rice cakes should be topped with apple wedges. They should be drizzled with honey and sprinkled with pomegranate arils.

52. Pumpkin Pie Spice Overnight Oats with Pear

Preparation time twelve hrs Cooking Time zero mins
Servings one person
Nutritional facts 223 calories Carb 35 gm Protein 11 gm Fat 5 gm Sodium 129 mg Potassium 377 mg
Phosphorous 150 mg
Ingredients

- Half fresh moderate pear
- Two third cup of unsweetened vanilla almond milk
- One third cup of old-fashioned oats
- A half teaspoon of pumpkin pie spice

Instructions

- Half a pear should be diced.
- In a mason jar, mix simultaneously all Ingredients and stir well. Refrigerate for around one night.
- The next day, it'll be ready to eat. Breakfast can be consumed on the go. It is not important to heat it. You may use a sweetener.

53. Oven Fried Fish

Preparation time fourteen mins Cooking Time twenty-five mins
Servings four persons
Nutritional facts 264 calories Carb 13 gm Protein 20 gm Fat 1 gm Sodium 67 mg Potassium 526 mg
Phosphorous 230 mg
Ingredients

- 2 teaspoons of Extra Spicy Blend (Mrs. Dash)
- 1/3 cup of corn meal
- one and a half tbsps. of lemon juice
- one to one and a quarter pounds of catfish or any other filets of white fish
- half tsp. of lemon zest, grated
- one and a half tbsps. of cumin
- 3 tablespoons of Mrs. Dash Garlic & Herb Blend
- 1 tablespoon of olive oil

Instructions

- Warm up your oven at 400 ⁰ F.

- Inside a small-sized container with a lid, mix olive oil, lemon juice, 1 tablespoon of Garlic and Herb, cumin, & one teaspoon of Extra Spicy.
- To blend the Ingredients, give it a good shake.
- Put the lemon juice mixture into a shallow container and coat the fish with lemon mixture on both sides.
- Mix Seasoning Blends, corn meal, and lemon rind inside a mixing container. To blend, mix everything simultaneously.
- Coat the fish on the both sides using the corn meal combination. You should bake for twenty to twenty-five mins, or till the fish easily flakes using a fork.
- If desired, serve with more hot pepper sauce and lemon juice.

54. Paella

Preparation time sixteen mins Cooking Time twenty-five mins
Servings six persons
Nutritional facts 233 calories Carb 25 gm Protein 20 gm Fat 2 gm Sodium 257 mg Potassium 40 mg Phosphorous 145 mg
Ingredients

- 1/2 pound of chicken breast, chopped
- one tbsp. of olive oil
- two jars of pureed roasted red peppers
- half lb. of Italian sausage
- half tsp. of Tabasco sauce
- half lb. of shrimp, shelled, uncooked, deveined
- two cups of short grain rice, uncooked
- half cup of frozen green peas
- half tsp. of paprika
- one and a half cups of chicken broth (low sodium)
- one-two pressed garlic cloves
- 10 strands or 1/8 teaspoon of saffron
- one cup of yellow onion, cut
- half cup of every green & red peppers, sliced in strips

Instructions

- Inside a big-sized pot, warm the olive oil & cook the chicken, sausage, as well as garlic till the meat is browned.
- Eliminate the meats from the pot and put them away.
- Sauté the onion and rice till the onion is transparent and the rice is light brown.
- Reflip the meat to the pot, along with the pureed red bell peppers and broth.
- Then the Tabasco, paprika, and saffron should be included inside a container.
- Get everything to boil, then flip down to low flame and cover for around ten mins.
- Include the bell peppers, shrimp, and peas and mix well.
- Cook for 10 mins with the lid on.

55. Pancit Guisado

Preparation time five mins Cooking Time fourteen mins
Servings six persons
Nutritional facts 287 calories Carb 39 gm Protein 19 gm Fat 5 gm Sodium 194 mg Potassium 391 mg Phosphorous 183 mg
Ingredients

- 1 pound of pork or chicken breast, boiled and sliced
- 1 tablespoon of diminished sodium soy sauce

- 8 ounces of rice stick noodles
- one cup of low sodium chicken broth
- half moderate sliced onion
- 1 sliced stalk celery
- 2 chopped green onions
- one and a half cups of green cabbage, shredded
- three cloves of garlic, crushed
- one lemon
- quarter cup vegetable oil
- one big carrot, peeled & sliced like the matchsticks

Instructions

- Rice noodles should be soaked in hot water for five mins prior to draining and setting aside.
- Inside a big-sized wok or griddle, warm the oil on moderate flame.
- You should sauté for around five mins with the garlic and onion.
- Mix the sliced cabbage, meat, and carrots inside a big-sized mixing container.
- It should be stir-fried for three mins.
- Chicken broth, low-sodium soy sauce, and celery are included to the pot.
- Cook for around three mins on low flame.
- Simmer for 3 mins after including the soaked rice noodles to the broth.
- Include the meat and veggie mixture to the noodles, garnish using green onions, and season using fresh lemon juice, if liked.

56. Parslied Onions and Pinto Beans

Preparation time nine mins Cooking Time twenty-five mins
Servings eight to twelve persons
Nutritional facts 458 calories Carb 78 gm Protein 26 gm Fat 5 gm Sodium 140 mg Potassium 207 mg Phosphorous 432 mg
Ingredients

- half cup of fresh dill
- one cup of Italian parsley, flat-leafed
- two tbsps. of butter
- half tsp. of curry powder
- 4 cups of pinto beans, low sodium
- 1 tablespoon of oil
- two cups of low salt chicken broth
- 6 cups of sliced onions
- one big lemon
- as required pepper
- 1 cup of curly parsley

Instructions

- Parsley and dill should be washed and dried.
- Remove any thick stems and slice into half to one-inch pieces prior to setting aside.
- Set the lemon aside after halving it and squeezing the juice.
- In a small-sized saucepot, mix the broth and halved lemon.
- Raise the broth to the boil. Afterwards, diminish to a low flame and cover to keep it warm.
- Warm the oil and butter inside a big-sized saucepot and cook the onions till they are wilted and golden.
- Include the parsley, curry powder, and dill inside a mixing container.

- Mix the broth and lemon halves inside a mixing container.
- Cook for a few mins to tenderize the parsley and diminish the broth mildly.
- Bring the beans & lemon juice to the boil and then remove from the flame.
- Lemon halves should be removed.
- You can season using pepper.

57. Hungarian Goulash

Preparation time fourteen mins Cooking Time one hr forty mins
Servings six persons
Nutritional facts 450 calories Carb 10 gm Protein 37 gm Fat 24 gm Sodium 200 mg Potassium 700 mg
Phosphorous 300 mg
Ingredients

- Two tsps. of sweet paprika
- two lbs. of beef round steak
- quarter cup of butter or oil
- One and a half cups of onions, sliced
- Quarter cup of flour
- 1 cup of low sodium beef stock
- One tablespoon of red wine or wine vinegar

Instructions

- Coat the meat in flour after cutting it into one-inch cubes.
- Brown the meat on both ends in a heavy pot with butter or oil.
- Whisk in the onion and cook for a few mins.
- Whisk in some stock. As needed, include more. It should have a thick, stew-like texture but be easy to stir.
- Conceal the pan with a cover.
- Cook the meat for around one and a half hrs on low flame.
- Eliminate the meat from the pot and keep it warm.
- Thicken with flour or corn starch after including paprika to the stock.
- Put in the vinegar.
- Serve goulash with salad and spaetzli or noodles.

58. Irish Baked Potato Soup

Preparation time fourteen mins Cooking Time, fifty-five mins
Servings six persons
Nutritional facts 275 calories Carb 39 gm Protein 14 gm Fat 27 gm Sodium 226 mg Potassium 800 mg
Phosphorous 261 mg
Ingredients

- Four ounces of cheese, cubed
- 2 big potatoes
- Four cups of skim milk
- A half teaspoon of pepper
- 1/2 cup of sour cream (fat free)
- One third cup of flour

Instructions

- Bake potatoes till tender at 400 $^{\circ}$ F till done.
- Allow to cool prior to cutting lengthwise and scooping out the pulp.

- Brown flour to a light brown color on moderate flame and then gradually include milk, stirring constantly till well mixed.
- Whisk in the potato pulp and season using salt & pepper.
- You need to cook, stirring frequently, over moderate flame till thick and bubbly.
- Mix in the cheese till it is thoroughly dissolved.
- Take the pot off the flame as well as stir in the sour cream.

59. Italian Meatballs

Preparation time nine mins Cooking Time fifteen mins
Servings twelve persons
Nutritional facts 163 calories Carb 4 gm Protein 13 gm Fat 32 gm Sodium 72 mg Potassium 199 mg Phosphorous 125 mg
Ingredients
- 2 big eggs, beaten
- 1/2 tablespoon olive oil
- half cup dry oatmeal flakes
- half teaspoon black pepper
- half cup sliced onion
- 3 tablespoons parmesan cheese
- 1.5 pounds ground beef
- one tsp. dried oregano
- half tablespoon garlic powder

Instructions
- Warm up your oven at 375 º F.
- Inside a big-sized mixing container, mix simultaneously all of the components and stir well.
- Put on a baking sheet and roll into 1″ balls.
- Then cook for around 15 to 20 mins, or till the meatballs are cooked.
- To serve, warm the meatballs in a warming dish or in a crock pot on low flame. It can be served with 2 teaspoons sauce.

60. Jammin' Jambalaya

Preparation time nine mins Cooking Time thirty mins
Servings six persons
Nutritional facts 200 calories Carb 19 gm Protein 16 gm Fat 2 gm Sodium 400 mg Potassium 314 mg Phosphorous 170 mg
Ingredients
- 1/4 teaspoon of cayenne pepper
- 7 ounces of sliced and smoked turkey sausage
- 1/2 big-sized yellow onion
- 2 teaspoons of olive oil
- half cup of rice (white or brown)
- half tsp. of dry thyme
- half tsp. of oregano
- one big chopped red bell pepper
- two bay leaves
- one two-third cups of chicken broth
- 1/4 teaspoon allspice
- three cups sliced collard greens
- 1/8 teaspoon of white pepper

- two minced garlic cloves
- quarter tsp. of black pepper
- half pound of jumbo shrimp, tails removed, cooked

Instructions

- Inside a big-sized griddle, warm the olive oil on moderate-high flame.
- Mix the onion, shrimp, collards, turkey sausage, bell pepper, and garlic inside a big-sized mixing container.
- You need to cook, stirring occasionally, for 10 mins.
- Bring the remaining components to the boil.
- Cover and cook for 20 mins, or till rice is tender, on moderate-low flame.

61. Kickin' Chicken Tacos

Preparation time twelve mins Cooking Time twenty mins
Servings four persons
Nutritional facts 141 calories Carb 9 gm Protein 14 gm Fat 9 gm Sodium 50 mg Potassium 220 mg Phosphorous 155 mg

Ingredients

- 1 1/2 teaspoons of salt-free taco seasoning
- one lb. of boneless and skinless chicken breasts
- two green onions (scallions), sliced
- 1 cup of iceberg lettuce, sliced or shredded
- quarter cup of sour cream
- one juiced lime
- half cup of sliced cilantro
- 8 corn tortillas

Instructions

- Boil the chicken for twenty mins at a low temperature.
- Chicken can be shredded or finely sliced into bite-size parts.
- Mix the Mexican seasoning, chicken, and lime juice inside a mixing container.
- Chicken and lettuce should be stuffed into tortillas.
- Sour cream, cilantro, green onions, or other garnishes can be included on top.

62. Kohlrabi Soup

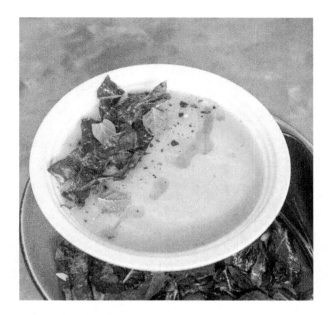

Preparation time nine mins Cooking Time thirty-five mins
Servings twelve persons
Nutritional facts 180 calories Carb 20 gm Protein 8 gm Fat 10 gm Sodium 200 mg Potassium 633 mg
Phosphorous 198 mg
Ingredients

- 2 quarts of low salt chicken broth
- Three pounds of kohlrabies
- 1 pound of celeriac
- One cup of light sour cream
- ground pepper as required
- one cup of chopped onions
- two tbsps. of butter
- half lb. potatoes
- a pinch of nutmeg

Instructions

- Kohlrabi, celeriac, & potatoes should all be peeled and chunked.
- Warm the butter in a big-sized saucepot as well as cook the onions till wilted, approximately 5 mins.
- Bring the vegetables and two quarts of broth to the boil and then diminish flame & simmer for around 25-30 mins, or till the vegetables are tender.
- Inside a mixer, puree some of the vegetables and broth till completely smooth; repeat till all of the veggies and broth are mixed.
- Reflip to the flame and stir in the pepper, cream, and nutmeg.
- If necessary, thin with more broth.

63. Lamb and Barley Casserole

Preparation time fourteen mins Cooking Time, three hrs twelve mins
Servings six persons
Nutritional facts 530 calories Carb 54 gm Protein 38 gm Fat 18 gm Sodium 137 mg Potassium 599 mg
Phosphorous 332 mg
Ingredients

- 2 moderate carrots, sliced finely

- 3 tablespoons of olive oil, divided
- Two moderate celery sticks, sliced finely
- 4 parsley sprigs, sliced
- 2 moderate onions, sliced
- 1 tablespoon of fresh thyme
- 6-8 lamb slices or lamb shanks
- 2 bay leaves
- one and a half cups of chicken broth (low sodium)
- two garlic cloves
- 1 cup of white wine
- 2 cups of barley

Instructions

- Warm up your oven at 300 ⁰ F.
- Take two tbsps. of oil and sauté garlic as well as vegetables till transparent and golden in a fry pot.
- Stir in the barley till it flips golden in color.
- Put in a casserole dish and bake.
- Prior to including the lamb to the casserole dish, brown it in a griddle.
- Put in the broth and season using herbs. If necessary, include more liquid to cover the barley.
- It should be baked for two & a half to three hrs in the oven
- When the barley is done, it should be mildly moist and the meat tender.

64. Lemon Curry Chicken Salad

Preparation time one hr ten mins Cooking Time zero mins
Servings four persons
Nutritional facts 276 calories Carb 15 gm Protein 15 gm Fat 1 gm Sodium 46 mg Potassium 221 mg Phosphorous 82 mg
Ingredients

- 1/4 teaspoon of ground ginger
- one and a half cups of grapes, halved
- quarter cup of vegetable oil
- one and a half cups of chicken, cooked & chopped
- one-eighth teaspoon garlic powder
- 1/4 cup of frozen lemonade concentrate, thawed
- half cup celery, sliced
- quarter tsp. curry powder

Instructions

- Whisk oil, lemonade concentrate, and spices inside a big-sized container.
- Rest of the Ingredients should be included and whisked mildly.
- It must be chilled for an hr.

65. Lentil meatballs or patties

Preparation time fourteen mins Cooking Time fifty-five mins
Servings eight persons
Nutritional facts 237 calories Carb 66 gm Protein 14 gm Fat 3 gm Sodium 242 mg Potassium 238 mg Phosphorous 161 mg
Ingredients

- two tbsps. of olive oil
- one cup of dried lentils

- 3 teaspoons Italian seasonings
- one pound crimini mushrooms
- 1/4 teaspoon of cayenne
- 3 crushed garlic cloves
- two cups panko breadcrumbs
- one cup parmesan cheese, shredded
- 2 eggs
- 1 moderate sliced onion

Instructions

- Four cups of water are to be included to one cup dried lentils in a saucepot. Raise to the boil and afterwards flip to a low flame and cook for around 15-20 mins, or till the potatoes are soft. Drain.
- Utilizing a mixing bowl or a knife, finely slice the mushrooms into 14-inch pieces.
- Include the oil and mushrooms to a frying pot and cook till the mushrooms are translucent. Cook for a few mins more after including the mushrooms and garlic.
- Insert all Ingredients inside a container as well as mash using a potato masher, or pulse several times inside a mixing bowl. You would like the mixture to be chunky rather than pureed. Stir in the remaining components till well mixed.
- To create meatballs, form 24 balls with an ice cream scoop. Form 8 patties, 4 inches wide and half inch thick, if making vegetarian patties. You could also create half the meatballs and half the patties and freeze half of them for another meal.
- Use a silicone non-stick mat or a baking sheet. Cooking spray or a tiny amount of the olive oil can be used to coat meatballs or patties. Warm up your oven at 400°F and bake for around 15 mins. Bake for another 15 mins on the other side.

66. BBQ Pineapple Chicken

Preparation time twelve hrs Cooking Time fifteen mins
Servings eight persons
Nutritional facts 140 calories Carb 23 gm Protein 10 gm Fat 2 gm Sodium 81 mg Potassium 253 mg Phosphorous 74 mg
Ingredients

- 1 tsp. of Dijon mustard
- Four oz. of skinless chicken breast, diced into two-inch cubes
- Two teaspoons of sliced garlic
- Half a teaspoon of wasabi paste
- Twenty oz. can of pineapple rings

Instructions

- Take the pineapple rings out of the can and keep the juice.
- Mix pineapple juice with mustard, wasabi paste, and garlic.
- Chicken breasts should be cut into 2-inch cubes.
- Chicken should be mixed with the pineapple juice mixture and marinated in the fridge for rest of the night.
- Place the chicken parts on skewers or cook them on a metal grate at the barbecue.
- Cook the chicken on a hot grill until it is cooked through and golden brown.

30-Day Meal Plan

Days	Breakfast	Lunch	Dinner
1	Strawberry and Peanut Oatmeal Container	Tilapia Tostadas with Corn-Zucchini Sauté and Basmati-Lime Pilaf	Fast Roast Chicken with Lemon & Herbs
2	Breakfast Quesadilla	Beef Thai Salad	Egg Fried Rice
3	Avocado Toast	Spicy Chicken Penne	Lamb and Barley Casserole
4	Blueberry Smoothie	Jamaican Steamed Fish	Confetti Chicken 'N Rice
5	Low Oxalate Granola	Vegetarian Red Beans and Rice	Low Sodium Sloppy Joes
6	Dilly Scrambled Eggs	Moroccan Chicken	Kohlrabi Soup
7	Spicy Tofu Scrambler	Asian Noodle Stir Fry	Paella
8	Loaded Veggie Eggs	Old Fashioned Canadian Stew	Grilled Salmon with Fruit Salsa
9	Apple Filled Crepes	Salmon Rice Salad	Mediterranean Pizza
10	Avocado Toast	Chicken Makhani	BBQ Pineapple Chicken
11	Maple Pancakes	Tuna Macaroni Salad	Crock Pot Chili Verde
12	Fresh Berry Fruit Salad with Yogurt Cream	Za'atar Chicken with Garlic Yogurt Sauce	Curry Chicken Salad
13	Banana Oat Shake	Eggplant and Tofu Stir-Fry	Pancit Guisado
14	Apple Bran Muffins	Fish Tacos	Jammin' Jambalaya
15	Pumpkin Spiced Applesauce Bread or Muffins	Kidney Bean and Cilantro Salad with Dijon Vinaigrette	Slow-Cooked Lemon Chicken
16	Southwest Baked Egg Breakfast Cups	Roast Beef with Yorkshire Pudding	Irish Baked Potato Soup
17	Fluffy Homemade Buttermilk Pancakes	Roasted Asparagus and Wild Mushroom Stew	Chicken, Red Pepper, Spinach and White Bean Pizza
18	Southwest Sweet Potato & Pineapple Hash	Baked Salmon with Roasted Asparagus on Cracked Wheat Bun	Cowboy Caviar Bean and Rice Salad

19	Renal-Friendly Homemade Sausage Patties	Rava Dosa: Low Sodium and Low Potassium Version	Beef Barley Soup
20	Apple Mint French toast	Green Garden Salad	Hungarian Goulash
21	Apple and oat cereal	Chicken in Mushroom Sauce	Dijon Chicken
22	Nutritious Burritos	Shrimp and Apple Stir Fry	New England Clam-Chowder
23	Egg and Sausage Breakfast Sandwich	Stir Fry Rice Noodles with Chicken and Basil	Honey Herb Glazed Turkey
24	Fruit & Cottage Cheese Omelet	Asian Eggplant Dip with Seared Peppercorn Steak	Chicken Lasagna with White Sauce
25	Yummy Omelet	Fish Cakes	Orange-Glazed Chicken
26	Banana-Apple Smoothie	Turkey Meatballs with Hot Sauce	Marinated Shrimp & Pasta Salad
27	Muffin Tin Eggs	BBQ lemon and dill salmon	Italian Meatballs
28	Lemon-Blueberry Corn Muffins	Crunchy Lemon Herbed Chicken	Mediterranean Roasted Red Pepper Soup
29	Chocolate Pancakes with Moon Pie Stuffing	Chicken and Gnocchi Dumplings	Honey Herb Glazed Turkey
30	Peach Raspberry Smoothie	Kidney-Friendly Chicken and Ginger Congee	Crock Pot White Chicken Chili

Conclusion

Salts and minerals in the blood are balanced by healthy kidneys. If you have (CKD) chronic kidney disease, your kidneys are unable to filter your blood properly. Your kidneys may be assisted by the things you eat and drink to maintain an appropriate amount of minerals and salts in your body, which actually leads to you for feeling healthier. This is because maintaining this balance will assist in helping your kidneys function properly. Consuming the right meals while preventing foods that are high in sodium, potassium, and phosphorus can help prevent or postpone the onset of some health problems that can be caused by CKD. The effectiveness of your kidney disease therapies may also be influenced by what you eat and drink. People with advanced CKD should be aware of how calories, lipids, protein, and liquids impact the body. To help you treat, manage and control your kidney function, you need to consume a balanced & renal-friendly diet. This book will not only help diminish the chances of kidney disease but will also help you in managing your kidneys function.